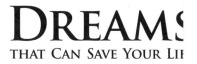

DREAMS
THAT CAN SAVE YOUR LIFE

D0204731

"This inspiring book could save your life or the life of someone you love. Dozens of medically verified stories of dreams accurately diagnosing, prognosticating, or suggesting the most effective therapies for deadly diseases will help you trust your dreams and intuition. Dreams are a vital part of the modern medical team. I rely on them. This book will convince you that you should, too."

— KATHI J. KEMPER, MD, MPH, author of *Authentic Healing*

"The authors provide the evidence we need to heed warning dreams. Live not in fear of them but in the joy of receiving the best of all gifts—a dream that can save your life."

— C. NORMAN SHEALY, MD, PhD, neurosurgeon and author of *Living Bliss*

"Information that comes to us through dreams can be important, compelling, and even lifesaving, as this beautiful book illustrates. Yet all too few of us are paying attention. Bravo to the authors for having the courage to step outside the medical box and expand our horizons. We are all enriched by their elegant work. They invite us to ask ourselves, 'What else is possible?' A life-changing question if there ever was one."

— THOMAS HUDSON, MD, radiologist and author of
Journey to Hope: Leaving the Fear of Breast Cancer Behind

"The most overlooked and neglected source of health information is our own unconscious mind, especially our dreams. This ancient, nocturnal avenue to wisdom is vividly described in *Dreams That Can Save Your Life*. These abilities are an inherent part of our nature. They are a magnificent gift. We ignore them at our own risk."

— LARRY DOSSEY, MD, author of *One Mind*

"This breakthrough book is the bridge we've all been waiting for that connects the metaphysical dream world with the practical world of medicine and science. After reading this book, you'll never again take your dreams lying down."

— KELLY SULLIVAN WALDEN, bestselling coauthor of
Chicken Soup for the Soul: Dreams and the Unexplainable

"This book not only contains case studies but tells its readers how to remember their dreams and put them to practical use. It needs to be widely read not only by physicians but by their patients. The authors have written a book that reads like a series of detective stories, with surprise endings that will motivate its readers to remember their dreams and take action on what they discover."

— STANLEY KRIPPNER, PhD, coeditor of
Working with Dreams and PTSD Nightmares

"This thrilling book combines the latest psychological research on the power of dreams to foretell the onset of cancer. The authors are awakening us to our innate power to perceive the reality of—and heal—our own lives and bodies."

— NAYASWAMI DEVI NOVAK, cospiritual director of Ananda
and corecipient of the Global Ambassador Peace Award
from the Institute of International Social Development

"The authors bring razor-sharp attention to one of the biggest epidemics of our times—cancer. Everyone would benefit from this eye-opening book. Read this book to know how dreams can work in conjunction with early diagnosis of diseases. This can make a big difference between suffering and healing, life and death."

— JERRY LAZARUS, author of *Dreams: Listening to the Voice of God*

"This very provocative book not only chronicles the predictive dreams of dozens of cancer survivors but also seems to activate such dreams within the reader. For anyone who wants to activate their own inner physician, I highly recommend it!"

— TRICIA McCANNON, author of *The Angelic Origins of the Soul*

"Reading the detailed narratives of the dreamers in these pages gives me hope for the restoration of dreams to their rightful place in medicine."

— JEAN-MARC EMDEN, CEO and cofounder of DreamsCloud.com
and cofounder of CircadiaLabs.com

DREAMS

THAT CAN SAVE YOUR LIFE

Early Warning Signs of Cancer
and Other Diseases

LARRY BURK, MD, CEHP

AND

KATHLEEN O'KEEFE-KANAVOS

Foreword by Bernie Siegel, MD,
author of *Love, Medicine and Miracles*

 FINDHORN PRESS

Findhorn Press
One Park Street
Rochester, Vermont 05767
www.findhornpress.com

Findhorn Press is a division of Inner Traditions International

Disclaimer
The information in this book is given in good faith and is neither intended to
diagnose any physical or mental condition nor to serve as a substitute for informed
medical advice or care. Please contact your health professional for medical advice
and treatment. Neither author nor publisher can be held liable by any person for any
loss or damage whatsoever which may arise from the use of this book or any of the
information therein.

A CIP record for this title is available from the Library of Congress

ISBN 978-1-84409-744-9 (print)
ISBN 978-1-84409-756-2 (e-book)

Printed and bound in the United States by Versa Press, Inc.

10 9 8 7 6 5 4 3 2 1

Edited by Nicky Leach
Cover design by Richard Crookes
Text design and layout by Damian Keenan
This book was typeset in Calluna and Calluna Sans.

To send correspondence to one of the authors of this book, mail a first-class letter
to the authors c/o Inner Traditions • Bear & Company, One Park Street, Rochester,
VT 05767, and we will forward the communication.

Contents

Acknowledgments

Kathleen (Kat) O'Keefe-Kanavos

Without the dedication, generous sharing of often very personal information and dream guidance of the following people, this book may not have been written, and a dream might still be considered "just a dream."

All of the women in Dr. Larry's Breast Cancer Dreams Project are amazing people and dreamers with whom it has been a pleasure to work and get to know on a personal basis. Suzanne De Gregorio painstakingly interviewed all the study group participants and helped write their stories. The dream study participants' stories are the backbone of the book. Suzanne's journalistic and editorial skills were a tremendous help.

Without the emotional support and understanding of my husband, Peter Kanavos, this book would not have been written. Many a night he made his own dinner and canceled "couple plans" so I could work into the wee morning hours to meet the book's deadline. Honey, I love you.

Working with radiologist and dreamer Dr. Larry Burk has been a dream come true. He is one of the easiest people in the world to collaborate with, and I feel privileged to have had the opportunity to be his co-author.

We also wish to honor Louise Hay of Hay House who died during the writing of this book (October 8, 1926 – August 30, 2017). Louise's groundbreaking New Thought and self-help ideals are embodied in this book.

Larry Burk, MD, CEHP

Discovering Kathleen (Kat) O'Keefe-Kanavos' incredible healing journey during my research was a tremendous gift from the dream world, and her enthusiastic energy propelled this book much faster than I could have imagined. My wife, Dagmar Ehling, supported me through the research and writing of the book and has been there every morning to share dreams with.

We would like to acknowledge Jean-Marc Emden, CEO of DreamsCloud, for his support of the Breast Cancer Dreams Project and the International Association for the Study of Dreams for promoting the research. Dr. John Palmer, of the Rhine Research Center, chaired the Institution Review Board that approved the research, and Drs. Christiane Northrup, Larry Dossey, and Lissa Rankin provided valuable assistance in recruitment of research subjects. Legendary dream researcher Bob van de Castle provided the inspiration for the project but died in 2014 prior to publication of the research.

Kat and Larry

A big "thank you" to our literary agent Devra Ann Jacobs, editor Nicky Leach, cover illustrator Richard Crookes, layout designer Damian Keenan, and publisher Thierry Bogliolo for believing in our project, and to all the other dreaming doctors, professionals, housewives, and total strangers who stepped forward and shared their amazing dream stories with us to not only make this book the best it could be but to save the lives of others.

Dream well.
Kat and Larry

Foreword

Bernie Siegel, MD

Dreams are the royal road to the unconscious.

— SIGMUND FREUD, *The Interpretation of Dreams*

I know how true the contents of this book are from my personal and professional experience. Consciousness speaks in dreams, symbols, and visions. The problem is that when our intellectual mind is controlling our thoughts and images, inner wisdom cannot break through the barrier and enter our conscious mind and awareness. I learned that during sleep or when in a trancelike state, in which we created images or heard voices speaking to us, our inner self was free to present us with the wisdom and truth the intellect blocked us from realizing.

Dr. Larry Burk, a radiologist at Duke University, just completed a groundbreaking study involving 18 women who had warning dreams preceding the diagnosis of breast cancer. This book contains their stories and the stories of other dreamers with dreams of different types of cancer and other illnesses that came true. These dreams involved spirit guides, angels, voices, tactile intervention in the dream, synchronicities, symbolism, and visitations from deceased loved ones. The dreams were all validated by a medical report.

I truly believe that the reason we sleep is not related to our need for rest but to our need to be in contact with the infinite wisdom available to our consciousness associated with past, present, and future life events.

After attending an Elisabeth Kubler-Ross workshop, in which she asked me to draw a picture for her, I became a believer. My drawing was an outdoor scene previously created in my mind to use in meditations. I handed it to her. She immediately asked me two questions: "Why is the number 11 important to you? And, what are you covering up?" I told her I had been working with cancer support groups for 11 months and was burying my painful feelings as a doctor about all the people I couldn't cure or help. I asked what made her ask those questions. She said there were 11 trees in the scene and I used a white crayon to make snow on a mountaintop when the page was already white. So, I had added a layer symbolic of covering something up.

It was incredible how much of my life was symbolically portrayed in a scene I thought had no meaning and was merely a matter of my imagination, but that experience made me go back to the hospital with a box of crayons and start to ask my patients to draw pictures for me, as well as share their dreams and intuitive wisdom. I was amazed at what I thought I was learning which no one else knew because this type of work is never a part of the information you receive while in medical school and training. An example is the fact that Carl Jung interpreted a dream and correctly diagnosed a brain tumor many years ago, yet I have never met a medical student who was told that while in school.

This book is important because it shows us the unity of mind and body, something the medical profession has a hard time dealing with. Many years ago, I put together an article on dreams and drawings and sent it to a medical journal for publication. It was sent back with the comment, "Interesting but inappropriate for our journal." So, I sent it to a psychology journal, and again it was returned, but this time the comment was, "It is appropriate but not interesting. We are aware of all this."

Healthcare practitioners and the general public need to access this wonderful source of wisdom, which can help in all phases of your life and is a gift from our Creator. Even the Bible shares that God speaks in dreams and visions. So quiet your mind and create the still pond that lets you see your true reflection, just as it let the ugly duckling realize he was a swan.

Based on people's dreams and drawings, I frequently made decisions as to whether they needed surgery or not and the best treatment for their disease. One woman with cancer said she had a dream in which a cat named Miracle appeared and told her which chemotherapy she needed to best treat her cancer. Her doctor agreed to do it, and she is alive and well. I named a kitten we adopted Miracle. She lived for 20 years.

Another woman whose story is in my book *A Book of Miracles* had a dark-skinned woman with an accent appear in her dream and tell her she had a lump in her right breast that needed to be looked into. She awoke from the dream and felt the mass in her breast. At the hospital, they diagnosed it as cancer and told her that the doctor who would be in charge of her treatment would be coming in a few minutes. When the door opened, in walked a woman doctor from India, the same person as in her dream.

On a personal level, at one time I was experiencing blood in my urine. My partners were all worried this was a symptom of cancer and urged me to get it checked right away. That night, while sleeping, I dreamt I was running one of our cancer support groups and asked everyone to introduce themselves and state why they were there. When it was my turn to speak, before I could utter a word, everyone said, "But you don't have cancer." As it turned out, I didn't.

And when I was questioning my ability to deal with and cope with death in a healthy way, versus denial of my mortality as a doctor, I dreamt I was a passenger in a car that went off a cliff. All the other passengers were screaming in fear while I sat back comfortable and relaxed, ready to accept my mortality and coming death. The looks I got from the other occupants were quite something.

My experiences with my patients, their dreams and mine are numerous. For me, there is no doubt or question that mind-body communication comes through dreams. They reveal our past, present, and future to us.

One thing that many art and psychotherapists miss is the anatomy that appears in dreams and drawings, as it was not part of their training. A jaundiced man drew a tree, which I knew revealed his bile ducts. I could see there was no obstruction in the ducts that would require surgery, and that the small ducts in the liver were blocked by an inflammation known as sclerosing cholangitis.

A woman who wondered whether she should have a mastectomy or a lumpectomy drew a tree with all the branches ending as if they had been pruned. It led her to say that the mastectomy was her right choice.

My mystic patient Monica, without any relationship or knowledge of my parents and patients, calls me with messages and knows the names of the people she is calling me about and I know the truth she speaks. When my mom died, the phone rang. It was Monica. "Your parents are together again and very proud of you, and they are being shown around by a lady who likes chocolate and cigarettes. Oh, it's Elisabeth Kubler-Ross showing your parents around." Yes, Elisabeth was my friend and teacher. Monica knows nothing of the events, but the infinite mind presents her with the truth to share with me, and allows us all to communicate with all living things that are conscious, from animals to people.

A lawyer I knew said, "I came to a conclusion that was eminently reasonable, totally logical, and completely wrong because, while learning to think, I almost forgot how to feel." What I have learned from my experience is that we are all multiple personalities. There is the thinker within us who does not always make the right decisions because, like the lawyer, they think and worry about what is correct while our unconscious and inner wisdom know what the right path to follow is and the choice for us to make. What I am about to share is my experience, and I believe what I experience. I am not blocked by preconceived beliefs or my inability to explain something.

The day my father was going to die, while I was out walking a voice asked me, "How did your parents meet?" I answered that I didn't know, and the voice said, "Then ask your mother when you get to the hospital." As soon as I walked into the room, that question popped out of my mouth. My mother answered, "Your father lost a coin toss and had to take me out." My father died laughing and looking fantastic because of my mother's stories. He didn't take his last breath until the last person who was coming that day entered the room. It was something he could not know, but it is just another coincidence of the wisdom and awareness of our dream state and consciousness.

I hear voices, see images, have visions and prophetic dreams, communicate with the dead and animals, and can be aware of the future and more. Yes, the child in me is ever open to new experiences. Many of these will be shared in the following pages to open your minds to our potential. We need to have a quiet mind to see the truth. Myths and fairy tales reveal this by using the still pond as the place to see your reflection and the truth about who you are: an ugly duckling or a swan.

I met my spirit guide while meditating and have had two people draw his picture and tell me he was standing beside me as I was lecturing and after a sermon at a friend's funeral. They saw him and described details no one could know who didn't truly see him. A third person even told me his name, which I knew from our original introduction to each other in my meditation. They helped me to understand that I was his voice and I have learned to let his wisdom flow through me as I speak.

Kathleen O'Keefe-Kanavos's profound story of dreams discovering her cancer, which was three times missed by the medical community and the tests on which they relied for early detection, yet discovered by her spirit guides in dreams, was shared on the *Dr. Oz Show* titled "The Sixth Sense: Shocking Premonitions." She wrote about her dreams in detail in her book *Surviving Cancerland: Intuitive Aspects of Healing*, in which pathology reports confirmed the diagnostic dreams.

One last point I would make is the importance of numbers in dreams and life. Our life's experiences are literally stored within us and revealed by numbers. When a reporter drew a picture with only one hand on a clock pointed at 12, and another woman drew a broken heart with 21 drops of blood, I asked them what happened when they were 12 and 21 and then heard their traumatic sexual abuse stories. I usually just question why the numbers portrayed are meaningful because they are not always traumatic events. They can be pleasant ones too, about family and life's joyful occurrences past, present, and future.

The research in this book focuses on precognitive dreams, which are capable of diagnosing an illness that is later medically validated. This book is filled with step-by-step advice and a collection of validated dreams that were true and amazing research.

Dreams can heal us. What used to be considered wishful thinking can now be validated by medical tests and pathology reports as seen by the numerous stories in this book. The research and personal experiences collected by Dr. Larry Burk and Kathleen O'Keefe-Kanavos prove dreams can come true, diagnose disease, and save lives.

The idea of dreams that diagnose disease and then come true is not new to the ancient world of healing, where dreams were shared with physicians and spiritual leaders as a window into truth. The fact that the dreams in this book are documented as being validated by current medical tests is groundbreaking evidence that dreams do have value in medicine. Let us hope medicine opens its mind, accepts the truth, and incorporates it into the process of healing versus focusing on a diagnosis and not the person with the diagnosis.

Closing this topic is hard to do because of all the stories I have to tell, from my dreams about *not* having cancer and not fearing death, to receiving messages through a mystic from dead family members and patients to hearing a voice speaking to me when my mind is in a quiet place. The messages were from my parents and patients and always entirely accurate and appropriate.

Folks, the mind is an amazing thing, and it and the body can communicate through dreams and symbols. So pay attention and listen to the wisdom of your dreams, psyche, and soma when they put on a show of images for you. They know what your consciousness is creating and planning for you because it knows what is the healthiest and safest path you should be taking with your life.

Preface

Larry Burk, MD, CEHP, and

Kathleen (Kat) O'Keefe-Kanavos

A dream, like every element in the psychic structure,
is a product of the total psyche.
— **CARL JUNG**, *CW 8, Para 527*

A vivid, more real-than-real dream that wakes you up and later comes true is one of the most awe-inspiring experiences a human being can have. It can be a life-changing event, especially when the dream is a compelling early warning sign of serious illness that leads to life-saving medical intervention. This unexpected intuitive information may actually prompt conventional diagnostic studies that turn out positive despite a lack of symptoms. The experience can create sufficient wonder at the mysterious workings of the universe to shake up the worldview of even the most conservative healthcare professional.

Fear of cancer is a common concern in our society, as evidenced by the many attempts to use technological screening tests for early detection with varying degrees of success and controversy. The inspiration for this book came from the first scientific study of dreams that warn specifically of cancer by Dr. Larry Burk, which included Kathleen (Kat) O'Keefe-Kanavos as one of the participants. "Warning dreams preceding the diagnosis of breast cancer: a survey of the most important characteristics," published in the 2015 May/June issue of *Explore: The Journal of Science and Healing,* reported the dreams of 18 women from around the world.

Since publication, we have been gathering reports of other similar breast cancer dreams, as well as warning dreams of many other types of cancer. These dreams cover the entire spectrum, including brain, colon, lung, ovarian, prostate, skin, testicular, tongue, and uterine cancers. Some of the dreamers also report continued use of their dreams for guidance and healing during therapy. We are hopeful that this preliminary research will inspire enthusiasm and funding for more rigorous studies to determine the evidence-based role of dreams in cancer screening, diagnosis, and treatment.

For those unfamiliar with dreams as they relate to health and dream interpretation in general, we will begin with a history of dreams in medicine in the Introduction. In Part One, we discuss the groundbreaking Breast Cancer Dreams Project. The incredible stories of the breast cancer dreamers will be presented in their own words in Part Two, with equally impressive dreams of other types of cancer in Part Three. After hearing these amazing stories, we hope you will be inspired to learn ways to enhance your own dream skills in Part Four. Other non-cancer, health-related dreams will be addressed in Part Five, and dreams for healing guidance will be included in Part Six. We are grateful to have a discussion of children's dreams by Drs. Kathi Kemper and Bernie Siegel in Part Seven. Intuitive dreams about other people's illnesses will be explored in Part Eight. Ideas about prevention, guidance, and spiritual implications will be summarized in the concluding Part Nine. The Appendices include a number of resources for your own dreamwork.

One of the most difficult tasks to pull off during these complicated times is open-mindedness. This is especially so when it comes to the importance of our dreams. The work shared in this book goes beyond preaching to the dream-choirs to enlighten and include anyone seeking a new perspective on the age-old subject of dreams that can come true and save lives. This book is common ground.

Let's be open-minded about yet unseen but dreamed possibilities. *Dreams That Can Save Your Life* spotlights exciting and new developments just outside the boundaries of the medical norm concerning dreams and illness. Imagine the possibilities of using dreams in the near future to predict or find earlier stages of disease not yet detectable by current medical tests.

This book, and the studies, stories, and dreams presented in it, authenticates a reality that is an integral part of everyday and every night life—our dreams. Which brings us back to our opening thought in writing this book: the need for open-mindedness concerning dreams that save lives.

The Cocktail Party Effect

Why do so many of the dreamers in this book hear their name called during the day, or at the end of a dream? This is known as the Cocktail Party Effect.[1] Experts in the field state that people are primed to detect personally significant words, such as names that have particular meaning to them and taboo words, such as sex, blood, death, cancer, dreams...[2] It may also describe a similar phenomenon that occurs when one may immediately detect words of importance originating from unattended stimuli, for instance, hearing a loved one's name in another conversation.[3]

This auditory phenomenon allows most people to "tune in to" a single voice and "tune out" all others, in a group, at a party, in a crowded place, or, in the case of this book, in a crowded dream.

It is also our hope that these dream stories create another phenomenon called Autonomous Sensory Meridian Response (ASMR).[4,5] It is an experience of "low-grade euphoria," when something important rings true and creates tingling that starts at the back of your head and travels down your arms and spine like you have been hugged by an angel.

Introduction –
The History of Healing Dreams

Larry Burk, MD, CEHP

Not infrequently the dreams show that there is a remarkable inner
symbolical connection between an undoubted physical illness and a
definite psychic problem so that the physical disorder appears as a
direct mimetic expression of the psychic situation.

— **CARL JUNG**, *CW 8, Para 502*

Dreams have provided useful information in medical diagnosis for cen-turies, beginning in ancient times with the shamanic traditions of the indigenous cultures around the world. Shamans dream intentionally for ailing tribal members as well as interpret dreams that occur during a healing crisis to provide therapeutic guidance.[6] Often dreams were responsible for instructing the shamans in the specific uses of medicinal plants. In *The Way of the Shaman,*[7] anthropologist-turned-shaman Michael Harner describes the phenomenon of the "big dream," which is "repeated several times in the same basic way on dif-ferent nights, or it is a one-time dream that is so vivid that it is like being awake, an unusually powerful dream."

In Native American tradition, vision quests involve four days and four nights of seclusion in nature seeking spiritual communication for guidance and insight. The Lakota word for vision quest is *Hembleciya,*[8] which translates to "Crying for a Dream." According to the legendary Lakota Holy Man Frank Fools Crow:[9] "My ancestors were all taught how to have sacred dreams. In these dreams, all kinds of strange and beautiful things would happen, things that never could take place in ordinary life. Strange beings would appear, and every kind of creature would come in impressive forms. These visitors would speak to the people and give them messages."

In ancient Greece, dreams were used in the Ascelpian temples for guidance on health-related matters, but this fact has been largely forgotten in mod-ern medicine.[10] There is great irony in this statement, as these temples were dedicated to Asclepius, the Greek god of medicine, whose rod with the single entwined snake is to this day the symbol of medicine.[11] Pilgrims would incubate dreams overnight in the temples and report them to a priest the next day, with the expectation of receiving an appropriate prescription for a cure. Particularly effective dreams might even provide a spontaneous healing by themselves. Dream incubation is a technique used to plant a dream-seed in the mind, in order for a particular dream topic to occur, either for recreation, love, health, or to attempt to solve a problem.

Centuries later, Sigmund Freud founded the field of psychoanalysis based on his dream work in psychotherapy, which included analysis of his own personal dreams.[12] His most famous dream report, about a patient named Irma in 1895, has been interpreted as being a foreshadowing of his death from mouth cancer diagnosed in 1923:[13] "She then opened her mouth properly and on the right hand I found a big white patch; at another place I saw extensive whitish gray scabs upon some remarkable curly structures which were evidently modeled on the turbinal bones of the nose. I at once called in Dr. M., and he repeated the examination and confirmed it."

Carl Jung, the founder of analytical psychology, stated, "I take dreams as diagnostically valuable facts," including their use in diagnosing medical conditions.[14] In discussing "big dreams," he noted:[15] "Looked at more closely, 'little' dreams are the nightly fragments of fantasy coming from the subjective and personal sphere, and their meaning is limited to the affairs of every day. That is why such dreams are quickly forgotten, just because their validity is restricted to the day-to-day fluctuations of the psychic balance. Significant dreams, on the other hand, are often remembered for a lifetime, and not infrequently prove to be the richest jewel in the treasure-house of psychic experience."

While these two pioneering psychiatrists were bringing dreams back into the realm of modern medicine, Edgar Cayce, The Sleeping Prophet of Virginia Beach, gave over 14,000 psychic readings in the first half of the 20th century, some of which included dream interpretation. Jerry Lazarus, an authority on Cayce's approach to dreams,[16] notes one reading specified that "Any condition becoming reality is first dreamed."[17] Another reading stated: "And too oft, ye disregard them; or too seldom do ye pay any attention to them! They are parts of thy experience. How often have you visioned in symbol or in dream those very things that happened to thee later!"[18]

Russian psychiatrist Vasily Kasatkin published the first research correlating dreams with physical illness in his book *The Theory of Dreams* in 1967.[19] An English report about this work was provided by Van de Castle.[20] Kasatkin based his observations on 10,240 dreams from 1,200 dreamers, most of whom had neuropsychiatric disease, including 44 cases of brain tumors and six cases of spinal cord tumors, as detailed in a translation by Susanne van Doorn.[21] He noted the following common dream features related to the presence of physical illness: 1) an increase in dream recall; 2) distressful, violent, and frightening images; 3) occurrence preceding the first symptoms; 4) long duration and persistence; 5) content revealing the location and seriousness of the illness.

English psychiatrist Robin Royston collected over 400 health-related dreams, including the case of a man who dreamed of a Black Panther digging its claws into his back at the exact site where his wife later discovered a mole that was diagnosed as melanoma. His story of "Bad Nancy" describes a dream play on words reported by a woman named Nancy who self-diagnosed her own breast "malig-nancy" in a dream of her pounding on her chest and shouting that accusatory name.[22] This dream and four others of women who dreamed about their breast cancers before diagnosis were described in detail in *Healing Dreams* by Marc Ian Barasch, including this observation by Royston: "These are not ordinary dreams, but big dreams, archetypal dreams, so laden with powerful emotional affect that the dreamer is forced to take them seriously."[23]

Barasch was motivated to research healing dreams by his own personal experience of dreaming his thyroid cancer diagnosis. Over a period of weeks, he experienced a series of ominous dreams focused on his neck culminating in one where "torturers had hung an iron pot filled with red-hot coals" under his chin. He was compelled to visit a physician who could find nothing wrong. The flood of nightmares continued until upon re-examination the doctor found a thyroid nodule. Biopsy showed a malignancy that was subsequently cured by successful surgery.

In the introduction to his book, Barasch outlines a multidimensional model for dream interpretation, which I have incorporated into my own approach. My guide to working with a dream diary by writing down a question before going to bed is summarized below and described in more detail with an illustrative dream example in the appendix of my book *Let Magic Happen: Adventures in Healing with a Holistic Radiologist*.[24]

1. Circle any words that seem to be unusual or out of place, and look them up in a dictionary to check for *wordplay* or unexpected *puns* related to your question.
2. Consider the dream from the *personal, shadow, warning, sexual, social, archetypal, synchronistic, and precognitive* perspectives.

3. Check for any *recurrent theme* from past dreams, and pay attention to any *animals* that visited you in the dream world.

4. Finally, ask yourself, *What does the dream want?* Give serious consideration to the possibility that the spirit world may have a question it wants you to answer in return.

5. *Sharing the dream* with someone who can provide candid feedback may provide a fresh perspective and additional insight.

Following this brief overview of the history of dreams in medicine, in Part One, we will share the inspiration for the Breast Cancer Dreams Project, Kat's story, a summary of the results of the project, a discussion of the dreaming e-patient, and basic dream categories.

PART ONE

Breast Cancer Warning Dreams

1

Origins of the Breast Cancer Dreams Project

Larry Burk, MD, CEHP

The greatest wealth is health.
— **VIRGIL**

The original inspiration for the research project that led to the publication of the "Warning dreams preceding the diagnosis of breast cancer" paper began in 2004, when Diane, one of my best friends, called me to say she had been diagnosed with breast cancer. A cardiac physiologist-turned-mindfulness meditation teacher, she had just had her 50th birthday and was previously in good health with no symptoms related to her breasts.

What Diane told me next would, many years later, send my research career off in an unusual direction—into the world of dreams. She said that a month earlier she had had a vivid, more-real-than-real dream of being on an operating room table having surgery on her breast for cancer by a woman surgeon. The dream was so compelling that she immediately went to her doctor to request a mammogram, even though she had no symptoms or a palpable lump.

After having the test every woman dreads, and sitting in the waiting room anticipating bad news, the woman radiologist came out to assure her everything was fine, and she could go home. Diane was so confident of the warning from the dream that she asked for an ultrasound just to be sure. The radiologist refused saying that since there was no lump or abnormality on the mammogram, she wouldn't know where to do the ultrasound exam.

Diane pointed to the spot indicated in her dream and refused to leave without the ultrasound being done in that location. The exasperated radiologist finally agreed and put the ultrasound probe on the spot. She was shocked to find a small cancer deep in the breast and turned white as a ghost. She stammered, "How did you know it was there?" Diane replied that she was shown the cancer in a dream, and as a radiologist, I can imagine that was quite an unexpected explanation for the doctor.

A referral to a surgeon for a biopsy led to another surprise for Diane. When she walked in the office, she recognized the woman surgeon from her dream, dramatically taking her precognitive experience to the next level. The future-vision scenario continued to play out in the operating room just as had been foretold in the dream, as detailed below in a summary from her dream diary in March and the narration of the scene in the operating room from April.[25]

> In March 2004, I had a vivid dream (unlike any before) in which I was lying on an operating table and a woman surgeon was operating on my left breast. At one point, she went to a microscope and looked through it and came back and told me that I have breast cancer. After hearing this news from the doctor, my daughter and former husband broke down and cried. I woke up.
>
> While I was startled, there was also a sense of calm at the same time; a knowing. I needed to get checked medically as soon as possible. An appointment was already scheduled several months later for my annual mammogram, so I called and moved it up.
>
> On April 9, 2004, I was lying on an operating table. A woman surgeon excised breast tissue, which was then examined under a microscope and determined to be cancer. Shortly after waking up from the anesthesia and getting dressed to go home, the doctor came to tell me that I had breast cancer. At home, my former husband and my daughter cried from the news.

We will return to Diane's remarkable story in Chapter 39, but for now let's just say I knew I had encountered an anomaly, kind of like when, in the movie *The Matrix,* Neo notices a black cat that appears near him on the staircase, then the scene repeats in identical fashion, representing a glitch in the program that runs the Matrix. Trinity and Morpheus react with alarm to his mention of this "déjà vu" experience, as it indicates a warning that something has changed in the program.

Eight years later, I was invited to present on a medical dream diagnosis panel at the annual Parapsychological Association meeting, held in Durham, NC, in August 2012. The other two panelists were Lori Fendell, a local acupuncturist/herbalist who dreams about her new patients the night before seeing them for the first time, and Jim Carpenter, a Rhine Research Center parapsychologist/clinical psychologist, who has dreams that guide him during his psychotherapy sessions.

After telling Diane's story, I was approached by Bob van de Castle, a famous dream researcher, about making a related presentation on dreams and cancer at the next International Association for the Study of Dreams (IASD) meeting in June 2013. Bob, along with Stanley Krippner, another legendary parapsychology researcher who was also in attendance at the meeting, had collaborated with psychiatrist Monty Ullman on the groundbreaking Maimonides dream telepathy research in the 1960s.[26]

At the same meeting, a physician/consciousness researcher friend of mine shared her story of breast cancer warning dreams with me, giving me reinforcement to submit the proposal to present at the IASD meeting. She had two scary dreams in one night, the first being about a serial killer, the kind that would make you get up in the middle of the night and check to make sure your doors are locked. The next one was about having breast cancer, which was found the next day on a mammogram without any symptoms.

It is a standard joke in medical research that when you discover one unusual diagnosis, you can say that you have "a case report." If you see another similar one, then you can say that you've seen "case after case." If you find a third, then you have "a series." The third one in my experience came from another friend who I had only met once during a week at a 2008 shamanic healing retreat in Brazil. Sonia Lee-Shield's story from her blog below is truly a cautionary one, which gave me the final push to do the research project.[27]

In Jan 2009, I had a dream that I had cancer. I went to the GP (general practitioner) complaining of a lump and spasm-like feelings on my sternum. The GP concluded it was normal breast tissue, and the feeling in my sternum was dismissed, a devastating mistake. A year later, a different doctor diagnosed stage 3 breast cancer. If there's one thing I could impart to everyone, it is that doctors and specialists make mistakes and when an inner voice starts screaming or dreaming you should listen.

Sonia died of breast cancer in 2013, and I now dedicate all my talks on this topic to her memory. Part of the motivation for doing research in this area is to make sure no other woman has her breast cancer warning dream dismissed by her doctor. Prompted by these dramatic tales of warning dreams, I decided it was time to do a literature search on breast cancer and dreams to find out if anyone else had ever heard of this phenomenon. Not surprisingly I found nothing at all in the mainstream medical literature.

The first relevant reference I found came from the dream literature; not a scientific one but a book by Wanda Burch, *She Who Dreams*.[28] Her book is a remarkable, skillfully narrated dream diary of her entire journey with breast cancer guided by a series of vivid dreams (see Chapter 13). In 1989, Wanda had intermittent pain in her breast with a question about a lump that could not be confirmed by mammogram or physical exam. Her dreams provided progressively more alarming images to this eventual climax.[29]

In 1990—after running the gauntlet of mammograms that denied the breast cancer I was dreaming fully by late November 1989, after the ultrasound in early 1990 that supplied only vague "wait and see" confirmation—I hounded my physicians until I was sent to a surgeon, Dr. Lyle Barlyn. I told him my dead father had made a dream appearance—after many disturbing nonspecific dreams—shouting that I had breast cancer and that I needed to do something about it now.

Dr. Barlyn asked, without flinching at the non-traditional source of my information, if I had dreamed the location of the tumor since it had not appeared on any of the medical tests. I had.

In a restless dream in between the terror of the possibilities implied in the "wait and see" ultrasound and my appointment with Dr. Barlyn, I had dreamed of a cone-shaped breast held in my hands. A stranger in the dream, unseen and to the side, asked that I turn the breast over. I saw a dark vial of liquid in a tube, and I saw its location. I took the breast and washed the dark liquid down the drain.

Dr. Barlyn listened to my dream and handed me a felt tip marker. "Draw the location on your breast." I drew a dot far underneath the right side of the left breast and told him that another dream had shown me a ledge, the dream debris—or tumor—hidden underneath the shelf. Dr. Barlyn inserted the biopsy needle in the area I designated and felt resistance, an indication of a problem. The surgical biopsy gave Dr. Barlyn the details of a fast-moving, incredibly aggressive breast cancer whose cells were not massing in a fashion that allowed them to be seen on a mammogram.

Despite the aggressive nature of the cancer Wanda's story has a happy ending which we will explore in Chapter 37. In 2004, when Wanda had recovered from the surgery and chemotherapy and written her book, she shared her dream stories with a local breast cancer support group at the Charles Wood Cancer Center in Glens Falls, New York. Surprisingly, 10 of the 19 women had warning dreams of their breast cancers, with dream visits from deceased family members in all but one of them.

Wanda's report was the tipping point for my interest in doing research on this topic, as it meant there must be dozens of women around the world who had experienced warning dreams. I wondered whether I had not heard anything about it before because women had not been telling their doctors about the dreams or whether their physicians were just dismissing them, as in Sonia's case. Was the concept just too far out to be accepted as valid in modern high-tech medicine?

The even more amazing phenomenon that Wanda and Diane experienced being able to exactly localize the breast cancers, as confirmed by imaging and biopsies, is the most paradigm-shifting aspect of the warning dream phenomenon for physicians. It is one thing to suspect that you have cancer as the result of a dream, but it is another whole level of information to be able to tell exactly where it is located. Author/internist Larry Dossey, MD, shared this additional example in his book *One Mind*.[30]

A woman had a dream that she had breast cancer. Worried sick, she visited her physician the next morning. She pointed with one finger to a specific spot in her upper left breast where she'd seen the cancer in the dream.

"It's right here," she said. She could not feel a lump, however, and neither could her physician. A mammogram was done, which was normal. When the doctor reassured her that nothing was wrong and that they should take a wait-and-see approach with frequent exams, she was not satisfied.

"This was the most vivid dream I've ever had," she protested.

"I'm certain I have breast cancer at this exact spot." When she insisted on going further, the physician, against his better judgment, pressured a surgeon to do a biopsy.

"But where? There's nothing there," the surgeon objected.

"Look, just biopsy where she points," the physician said.

In a few days, the pathologist called the original doctor with the report.

"This is the most microscopic breast cancer I've seen," he said. "You could not have felt it. There would have been no signs or symptoms. How did you find it?"

"I didn't," he replied. "She did. In a dream."

When Dr. Dossey heard that I was considering doing research on this topic, he told me about Carolyn Kinney, a retired nursing professor who had published a 1996 paper in the nursing literature about her personal account of having a warning dream.[31] She had a maternal history of breast cancer and was woken up by a commanding dream message. "Go make your appointment for your mammogram right now. Do not delay." Despite a lack of symptoms, it was confirmed by mammography and surgery. She tells more details about her story in Chapter 12.

When I gave my presentation on Dream Diagnosis of Cancer and Clinical Correlation at the IASD meeting in Virginia Beach, my initial dream teacher, Marcia Emery, was the moderator. She surprised me by saying, "I am 75 years old and have never had a mammogram in my life. I trust that if I am ever going to get breast cancer, I would have a dream about it first." As a radiologist, I wouldn't feel comfortable recommending such an extreme position, but it got the talk off to an auspicious start.

In the audience at the presentation was Bob van de Castle who shared his own personal story about having received warning dreams about his own rare cancer, an angiosarcoma of the face, years ago. Also in the audience was Jean-Marc Emden, CEO of DreamsCloud, the social networking site for dreams. He participated in a lengthy discussion period after the talk, during which we brainstormed on how to design a study about breast cancer dreams and he offered to be a sponsor for the research.

The final piece in the research project development came later that summer, when I discovered Kat's stories about her warning dreams. I was thrilled to hear that her book, *Surviving Cancerland: Intuitive Aspects of Healing*, had been published with an endorsement from one of the first physicians I had ever heard give any credibility to dream guidance: Dr. Bernie Siegel, author of *Love, Medicine and Miracles*. The next chapter will provide you with a through-the-looking-glass adventure into Kat's Alice in Wonderland world of intuitive dreams.

2

A Feather for Your Dreams

Kathleen (Kat) O'Keefe-Kanavos

*"Everyone dreams. Some dreams change lives. Other dreams save lives.
Validation is the key."*

NOTE: This chapter is adapted from my book *Surviving Cancerland:
Intuitive Aspects of Healing*. The names of the doctors in my story
have been modified to respect their privacy.

As a Special Forces army brat, born, raised, and educated in Europe, challenges, changes, and uncertainty were a part of my daily life. If we were lucky, my father only transferred to a new military base every two years. When we were unlucky, I attended five different first grades.

Shortly after transferring from Bad Toelz to Berlin, Germany, in 1961, the Berlin Wall separating East Berlin and West Berlin was built... overnight. The ensuing chaos was bloody and deadly. When I returned to the United States for the first time in order to attend college, I was a stranger in my own land. But nothing, except my dreams, prepared me for the fight of my adult life: cancer.

The Fight for My Life

The year is 1998, and I am in Boston, Massachusetts, with my gynecologist and general practitioner, Dr. Dennis Wagner, who resembles the late actor Gary Cooper. A guided dream from the previous night involving a Franciscan monk has sent me to his office for an examination. This is the first of many medical visits we will have over the next three months.

When Dr. Wagner enters the examining room, the theme song from *High Noon* plays in my head. "I can't feel anything on or around your breast, Kathy."

Torn between relief and concern, I wonder if the tiny spot is absent or if he has missed it?

"Perhaps you felt a fibrous tumor sensitive to your menstrual cycle. Let's do another mammogram and keep an eye on it. You're only 43, too young for breast cancer, you know. Go home. I'll call you with the mammogram and blood test results. And, I'll see you in six months," he concludes and snaps my chart shut.

If he isn't worried about this invisible hard spot, why am I? After all, he's the doctor, right? But the voices from my dream world refuse to be silent in my waking world and nag my every thought. *Go back to your doctor,* they keep saying.

My life has always been active and healthy. But three mammograms, three blood tests, three physical exams, three yellow copies of healthy mammogram reports over a three-month period, and three recurrent lucid diagnostic and prophetic dreams with Franciscan monks would send me scurrying back to my doctor. After my final healthy mammography report, I had this dream.

The Franciscan Monks

While enjoying my dream, it suddenly stops, like a frozen computer screen or a TV show put on pause. In the center of my dream a pop-up window appears, much like on a computer. The window expands into a door, and a spirit guide/ guardian angel dressed as a Franciscan monk in a long, brown, hooded robe with a knotted-rope belt and leather sandals steps through the Sacred Dream Door. His hood covers his face. "Come with me. We have something to tell you."

Am I dreaming in a dream, I wonder, but obediently followed him into a room I call the Room Between Realms, a place that is neither of the living nor the dead. It is a parallel universe of consciousness. Waiting for me are two other monk guides. A monk takes my hand, places it on my right breast, and says, "You have cancer right here. Feel it?" I did. "Go back to your doctor tomorrow without an appointment."

I start to cry and tell him that the doctors won't listen to me tomorrow any more than they did yesterday. "They just keep giving me the same tests over and over and tell me I'm healthy. If you want me to live, you help me."

My guide reaches into his enormous sleeve, pulls something out, and hands me a tiny white feather, no larger than one that escapes from a pillow at night and glides to the bedroom floor.

"Use this feather as a sword to fence within your verbal battles with the doctors, and you will win against scientific facts. You need exploratory surgery. If you present your case to the doctors as though you were an attorney standing before an incredulous judge who dislikes you, you will win," he says, then turns and walks out of my dream.

The Sacred Dream Door closes behind him, and my previous dream starts back up right where it had stopped, as if someone had taken it off pause.

Time had stood still as the monks from beyond time and space delivered their life-saving message in this esoteric dream-plane.

Reaching Critical Crossroads

Do I believe my doctors or dreams? Should I tell Dr. Wagner about the monk and the feather? My goal is to get help, not a padded cell. But, I returned armed with my feather.

Dr. Wagner looks at me as though I have just set myself on fire. "You want exploratory surgery! I can't take something out that isn't there." My doctor is upset. So am I, but for a different reason. His concern is I've overreacted to an "imagined spot." Mine is I haven't reacted enough to this damned dreamed spot.

As a doctor, he is armed with tangible, indisputable medical evidence in the form of mammography and blood test results from one of the top medical facilities in the world. I'm armed with an imaginary angel feather from a monk in a dream. *Oh, Lord have mercy! Did I really just think that? I want to take my feather and go home now. I'm taking a giant leap of faith here, so dreams and God, please don't let me down!*

I silently pray, then dig into my mental war chest, pull out the tiny angel feather, mentally pinch it between my fingers, and turn to face my medical opponent, who must become an ally. I take careful aim and plead my case. "I know something's not right. Prove me wrong."

"At 43 years of age you are too young for breast cancer, and it does not run in your family. I think if anything is there it is just a fibrosis tumor," he said.

"Who is going to do the surgery? And shouldn't we have an oncologist present?"

"No, I'll do the surgery. You do not have cancer."

"Okay, let's close her up."

Dr. Wagner's voice echoes down a dark tunnel of black, drug-induced dreamland, where I've been floating in suspended animation during surgery. I claw my way toward consciousness, light, and sound.

"What is it?" I ask, dragging myself over the precipice of anesthesia.

Eyes above masks fly open as medical personnel stare in disbelief. "Did she just speak?" a voice asks from above my head. I gaze up at someone peering down. Thankfully, the anesthesiologist blocks the overhead light.

"It's... it's just what we thought, Kathy—a fibrosis tumor," Dr. Wagner stammers, still frozen in shock, gloved hands held high, eyes wide as if seeing a ghost.

The overwhelming pain in my breast hits me, causing me to groan.

"Give her more anesthesia... now!" are the last words I hear as I slide back into the dark rabbit hole of anesthesia and resume floating in suspended black nothingness.

The First Cancer Warning Bell Tolls in My Waking Mind

Dr. Wagner pulls the privacy curtain behind him in the recovery cubicle, and my first warning bell rings. The second bell gongs when he takes my hand.

"Pathology didn't like what they saw when they opened the tumor," he says. Panic replaces my nausea. "Is it cancer?"

"Yes, I'm sorry. I'll refer you to a specialist now."

So my diagnostic dreams had been right: the tests were wrong.

My surgeon's words are the first shots fired in an ensuing battle. They are not warnings fired across my bow; they are point-blank into my breast. I glance down at my painful wound and weep.

Thus begins my descent down the dark rabbit hole of Cancerland. Like Alice, I'm falling, falling through a disturbing nightmare with no bottom in sight and little hope of landing softly. Oh, God! I think I'm in big trouble. My dreams had prepared me for what pathology had just validated. I have cancer! The dreams that drove me crazy also spurred me to action, and I hope saved my life. I focus on that positive thought but cry louder.

Scared out of my mind, I realize how much I need my dreams. Winning this war will require a viable weapon beyond the medical community. Had I not been a squeaky wheel, I'd be dying right now. Hell, I might be dying anyway. What a kick in the pants that would be.

But my dreams had armed me with a powerful feather once. Perhaps the monks have more where that one came from if I need them in the future. If I still have a future. With that thought, I stop crying and slip into an exhausted, dreamless slumber. The feather had won out over hospital policy. The exploratory surgery discovered the foretold lump. The first pathology report stated it was hormone-receptive stage 2 aggressive DCIS ductile carcinoma in situ. A second surgery was required by an oncologist to check for clean margins. Cancer was found in a lymph node.

Dr. Larry Burk's Dream Study

During the course of a Whole Life Expo event in Los Angeles where I was speaking about dreams that come true, I was told by a colleague about Dr. Larry Burk and his research on dreams that come true.[32] I called him up, we spoke, then became guest bloggers on each other's blogs, which were also published on DreamsCloud.[33]

A year later, we presented together on warning dreams at the International Association for the Study of Dreams (IASD) in San Diego. The story of how precognitive dreams can save your life and Dr. Larry Burk's research project was shared in February 2017 on *The Dr. Oz Show* episode entitled "The Sixth Sense: Shocking Premonitions."[34]

My cancer treatment was Adriamycin Cytoxan chemotherapy, radiation, and Tamoxifen. The dream validation was surgery and a pathology report. But, this is only the first of many dreams about cancer that came true...

KAT'S DREAM INTERPRETATION

Many dreams intersect or contain multiple categories, as described in detail in Part One. This is a lucid, recurring, precognitive, diagnostic (subcategory of literal and active) dream that does not require researching signs and symbols because it is so literal through conversation. It is precognitive because it tells me if I use the feather as a sword in my waking world, I will get the tests I need to find cancer. It is lucid because I know I am dreaming; active because the Franciscan monks in the dream placed my hand on my breast and handed me a talisman in the form of a feather; and diagnostic because it is validated by pathology reports. However, it contains some incredible symbols to reinforce the message.

A *Franciscan monk* is a positive symbol of spirituality. Monks are solitary in order to condition and align their mind and body with spirit and God. To dream of a monk may mean the dreamer should separate from worldly distractions and look within for answers through self-examination (a play on words for cancer) to achieve inner balance.

A *white feather* is a symbol of power, faith, truth, and protection in many dream cultures and is typically seen as a sign from an angel or passed-over loved one. A feather offered as a sword is a spiritual protection to win a battle. In my case the fight was two-fold: win against the doctor's arguments not to do more testing, and ultimately to win the war against cancer by trusting in spiritual guidance from within. In ancient Egyptian mythology, the white feather symbolized truth. Upon death, the god Osiris placed the heart of the soul on a golden scale against a white feather. If the soul was lighter than a feather, the soul was admitted into afterlife bliss. On a figurative level, my dream was saying spiritual guidance and truth will overcome all obstacles. In a literal translation, my dream said, *You have cancer, and if you fight using truth and spirituality, you will win.*

DR. BURK'S COMMENTARY

Kat's book, *Surviving Cancerland*,[35] is full of amazing stories of dream guidance through an Alice in Wonderland world of miraculous diagnosis and healing, like the scene on the book cover. It would be great if everyone could gain access their "inner white feathers" during their healing journeys, and as she describes, dreams are an excellent way to do that. You may not get a robed Franciscan monk as a guide, but as the stories of the other breast cancer dreamers in the next chapters illustrate you may get just what you need for your personal situation. Fasten your seat belts for an amazing ride stepping through the looking glass into the realm of dream diagnosis.

3

Warning Dreams Preceding the Diagnosis of Breast Cancer Research Results

Healing comes only from what leads the patient beyond himself and beyond his entanglements in the ego.

— CARL JUNG, *CW 13, Para 397*

The first step in the Breast Cancer Dreams Project was to get Institutional Review Board (IRB) approval to do research on human subjects. Since I had been a previous board president of the Rhine Research Center in Durham, NC, their IRB, which was run by respected parapsychologist John Palmer, was the best choice for a dream study that might include information about ESP and precognition. Dr. Palmer was quite helpful in making sure that the research complied with appropriate ethical and scientific guidelines.

Following IRB approval, the next step was to obtain a small amount of funding—$72, to be exact, for a subscription to SurveyMonkey—to create the breast cancer dreams survey questionnaire. By way of contrast, major breast cancer imaging studies of mammography, ultrasound, or magnetic resonance imaging (MRI) usually cost thousands of dollars and are often funded by the National Institutes of Health (NIH), Susan G. Komen, or the Dr. Susan Love Research Foundation. The latter two institutions declined to support the dream study because I did not have an NIH grant.

Fortunately, DreamsCloud, the online public platform for dreams sharing via social network, was willing to provide the small amount of funding and publicity needed to assist in recruiting research subjects who had dreams prior to diagnosis that would qualify them for the study. DreamsCloud created a page on their international website to launch the project and a platform for the survey. I also promoted it extensively through social media, with assistance from the International Association for the Study of Dreams and Drs. Christiane Northrup and Lissa Rankin.

It was actually much harder to find the breast cancer dreamers than I thought it would be, as unfortunately, I could not get a single breast cancer support group to participate in the research. It turns out that the tight-knit community of breast cancer patients and the healthcare providers who work with them is a closed circle when it comes to outsiders from other specialties like me. This is too bad, as the Dr. Susan Love Research Foundation has over 380,000 volunteer research subjects in its Army of Women.

I realized then how important it was to get a small pilot project published in a legitimate medical journal to provide a solid scientific platform for future more ambitious and well-funded projects that might be able to appeal to this much larger pool of participants. We launched the survey during Breast Cancer Awareness Month in October 2013, complete with a pink ribbon. The study closed at the end of March 2014, after 18 women from around the world completed the survey.

The 19 yes or no questions in the questionnaire are listed below:

1. Did you have any dreams warning about breast cancer before your diagnosis?
2. Do you keep a dream diary to record your dreams?
3. Did the first clues about the breast cancer come in your dreams?
4. Did you have more than one dream warning you about breast cancer?
5. Did the dreams increase in intensity, specificity, or urgency with time?
6. Were the dream(s) more vivid, real, or intense than your ordinary dreams?
7. Did the dream(s) contain an emotional sense of threat, menace, or dread?
8. Were the specific words "breast cancer" or "tumor" used in the dream(s)?
9. Did the dream(s) localize the tumor to a particular breast and specific location?
10. Did the dream(s) involve the sense of physical contact with your breast?
11. Did you receive a breast cancer dream message from a deceased family member?
12. Was there a sense of conviction about the importance of the dream(s)?
13. Did the dream(s) prompt you to seek medical advice and diagnostic testing?
14. Did you share the dream(s) with your doctor?
15. Did the dream(s) directly lead to the diagnosis being made?
16. Did you ignore the dream(s) until the diagnosis was made for another reason?
17. Did you forget about the dream(s) until after the diagnosis was made?
18. Did you overlook the significance of the dream(s) until after the diagnosis?

19. Did anyone else you know have dreams warning about your breast cancer?

We also asked the women in the study to write a narrative of their dream experiences to supplement the questionnaire. Unfortunately, Sonia Lee-Shield died before she could complete the survey. However, the rest of the women from Chapter 1 all participated along with other women from the United States and Great Britain, as well as Austria and Columbia. Two other women also responded but were not included because one dreamed only about a recurrence, and one turned out to have benign disease.

The survey was published in *Explore: The Journal of Science and Healing* in 2015.[36] The most common five characteristics of warning dreams in descending order of frequency were: a sense of conviction about the importance (94 percent); more vivid, real, or intense than ordinary (83 percent); an emotional sense of threat, menace, or dread (72 percent); the use of the specific words "breast cancer/tumor" (44 percent); and the sense of physical contact with the breast (39 percent).

In more than half of the cases, the women shared dreams with their doctors that indicated the locations of the cancers, leading directly to a diagnosis. Warning messages from deceased family members were far less frequent than we would have expected, based on Wanda's previous informal survey from 2004 described in Chapter 1. However, there were dream messengers in a quarter of the dream stories, often a doctor wearing a white coat, although other more metaphysical characters also appeared, such as Kat's monks.

More than half of the women kept dream diaries providing detailed narratives and dates for the dreams. A third of the time, the importance of the dreams was not appreciated until the diagnosis was made for another reason. In a quarter of the cases, there were multiple warning dreams increasing in intensity with time. The woman whose only warning dream occurred at the time of her second recurrence woke up with the question, "Where is it?" and found a lump hidden in her armpit.

The woman who turned out to have benign disease had a dream similar to the others, prompting the need for more research to differentiate benign versus malignant dreams.

A man illuminated in white light held up a glowing pearl and showed it to me. He said, "You have breast cancer. It's in your left breast, close to your chest wall. It is this size. You need to have it checked out."

She assumed it was malignant, but after 18 months of energy healing, she eventually had a benign adenoma removed at surgery.

In fact, there actually is evidence that some cancers may regress over time.[37] One of the criticisms of our survey study is that there was no control group of women with such benign disease. Since about a third of suspicious lesions on mammography turn out to be malignant at biopsy, there is an opportunity to do a more sophisticated research project focused on dreams of women who undergo biopsies. That way we will get information about the dreams of the other two-thirds of women with benign disease.

Two sisters in the study have a family history of breast cancer and carry the BRCA gene. The 12 percent lifetime risk of breast cancer in the general population increases to 45 percent with the BRCA2 mutation and to 65 percent with the BRCA1 mutation.[38] Up to 25 percent of hereditary cases of breast cancer are due to a mutation in one of these rare genes that code for tumor-suppressor proteins.[39] Four other women also shared that they had a family history of breast cancer without mention of genetic testing.

Prior to the development of radiological imaging techniques, having a positive family history was the only way to predict an increased risk of breast cancer. The National Cancer Institute (NCI) estimates that in 2015 there were 232,000 women newly diagnosed with breast cancer and 40,000 breast cancer deaths with 89 percent surviving five years.[40] Mass population screening mammography was introduced in the 1960s in an attempt to detect cancer in women prior to the onset of symptoms.

This approach has been called into question through an ongoing debate about the risks and benefits of mammography.[41] In 2009, the U.S. Preventive Services Task Force (USPSTF) published recommendations for routine screening every two years starting at age 50[42] in conflict with the current ACR recommendations for screening every year starting at age 40.[43] Women who follow the USPSTF guidelines should consider starting mammography earlier if guided by their dreams.

In high-risk women with the BRCA genes, magnetic resonance imaging (MRI) is recommended as an additional screening method. MRI is particularly useful for women with dense breasts where mammography has a more difficult time finding cancer.[44] Ultrasound can also be helpful in finding cancers in women under the age of 50 with dense breasts.[45] In women with a positive family history who cannot undergo MRI, ultrasound may be used as a supplemental screening test. Thermograms are performed noninvasively using a digital infrared camera. Thermography may detect some cancers before mammography, but may also miss cancers detected by mammography making the two approaches potentially synergistic in screening. Typical breast thermograms are symmetrical and stable over time on follow-up examinations, and the development of a positive asymmetric pattern is considered to be a high-risk factor for breast cancer.[46]

With all these technological options and conflicting opinions, it is a timely opportunity to consider using a dream diary as a supplement to breast self-examination, especially for high-risk women. The results of this study can empower women to feel more comfortable sharing their dreams with their doctors. It also offers a foundation for future research to determine the frequency of such dreams in women without known breast cancer in order to assess the predictive value of a warning dream.

4

The Rise of the Dreaming E-Patient

In the 1970s, the phrase "e-patient" was born.
In the ensuing decades, it grew up a bit, developing and building
its catchphrase," equipped, empowered, and enabled."
— **RICHARD DAVIES DEBRONKART JR.**
aka e-patient Dave/cancer patient

Much as dreams are windows into another information dimension; the internet is a type of informational Universal Wisdom Window at our fingertips. Access to the internet has created a new type of patient: the e-patient.

Many of the dreamers in the book are e-patients. It is how many of us found each other, Dr. Larry Burk's Breast Cancer Dreams Project, and the groundwork that led to this book.

According to Wikipedia, the e-patient is an individual or health consumer who participates fully in his or her medical care. The dreamer e-patients in this book combined dream information with internet information to fully arm themselves with facts for their life-saving journey back to the path of health and wellness. Prophetic dreams plus internet information created a powerful weapon to combat illness.

The late Dr. Tom Ferguson coined the term e-patient. He was a pioneering physician, author, and researcher who studied and wrote about the empowered medical consumer and the online health resources for consumers.[47] According to Dr. Ferguson, the e-patient is Equipped, Enabled, Empowered, and Engaged in their health, healthcare decisions, and choice of healthcare professionals and systems that support them.

E-patients see themselves as equal partners with their doctors in the healthcare process and are a new big wave in the ocean of internet users. This new type of patient gathers information about medical conditions that impact them and their families by using digital tools for research.

The dreamer e-patients in this book validated their dreams with internet content to get the treatments they knew they needed to survive illnesses. These dreamers used the internet as a health resource, studying up on their own

41

diseases, and those of friends and family members, to find better treatment centers, doctors, and to insist on better care.

They also used their experiences with dreams, healing, and internet research to provide other patients with invaluable medical assistance and support. The dreamer e-patients in Dr. Larry Burk's study group have increasingly served as important collaborators and advisors for their peers. They have documented their personal journeys on social media sites, online magazines, Internet TV sites, blogs, and forums. They foster an open dialog via comments and offer support to those who need it (see individual bios in the back of the book for further information on contacting contributors).

If our dreams were not meant to help us overcome a life-threatening illness, would we have had precognitive dreams that came true and saved our lives? If our illness were to be our "exit strategy," as Dr. Larry Burk calls it, we would have simply finished our days in blissful ignorance, rather than living the daily nightmare of convincing disbelieving medical personnel that we needed additional tests on what cannot be seen with the naked eye or certain medical tests, or felt... only dreamed. The proof is in the pathology reports.

Despite the slow responses to dreams or researched suggestions from patients, this is not a doctor-slamming book by any stretch of the imagination. Doctors do the best they can with what they have available to them, and what they have been taught. As Dr. Bernie Siegel explained in an internet TV interview with Dr. Larry Burk on the *Kat Kanavos Show*, titled "The Gift of Diagnostic Dreams in Medicine":

> Larry and I got information in medical school; we didn't get an education.
> Doctors don't get into people's lives to see what makes them vulnerable, which may be part of the cause of their physical disease. When Larry and I were in medical school, we were trained to treat the result, not the cause of illness.
> I have been working with dreams—for a hundred years or so—and believe if we listen to our dreams they will correctly diagnose our life. I don't know of any medical schools that tell their students to ask people what they are dreaming.

However, without the time and treatment recommended by our doctors, many of us would not be alive to share our stories in this book, including the parts about how we researched our dreams as e-patients. Although they did not know it at the time, our doctors were a part of our dream team.

From the physician's perspective, there is a standing joke about patients getting second opinions from Dr. Google. There are pros and cons to this issue.

Fortunately, patients who do their own research can be much better informed and equipped to participate in their own care. Unfortunately, most doctors only have a limited amount of time to explore the overwhelming amount of information available on the internet that is relevant to each individual patient, so being presented with a stack of printed-out material during a short office visit is often not well received. The new generation of cyber-savvy doctors is probably better able to cope with this data overload, although being younger does not give you longer appointment slots.

5

Basic Dream Categories

Physician, heal thyself.
— LUKE *4:23. 23*

Prior to delving into the stories of the dreamers from the Breast Cancer Dreams Project in detail in Part Two, we want to give you a way to understand the different types of dreams you will encounter there and in your own dream life. How often have you awakened confused, elated, or wondered what sort of bizarre dream you just experienced? And if dreams are unimportant, meaningless, mental mumbo-jumbo why do we, and all other living creatures, spend about one-third of our lifetime dreaming?

Although experts agree that there are numerous categories and sub-categories of dreams, this book will focus on the seven most basic groups, their meanings, and how to recognize and use them for life, love, wealth, and health.

This chapter defines dreams in easy-to-remember classifications. Yes, you can dream your life to wellness. The key is remembering your dreams, briefly covered in the Introduction, and will be explored in greater detail in Part Four. After you have recalled and saved your dream in a journal, identify it by using the information below. Then look for validation within the dream to be sure you defined it correctly.

Daydreams

Daydreams are mental wanderings or meanderings without a purpose. You are awake but no longer focused on a task. They also happen when you are bored. Have you ever found your mind drifting off into imagery and experiences like flying through the air or fighting an imaginary foe? You may be taking a break from stress or everyday life in order to solve a problem, build self-esteem, make plans for your future, or allow time and space for creativity.

Daydreaming is an ordinary form of altered consciousness concerning what is happening around and in your life at all times. Consciousness is your level of alertness during your waking hours. Daydreams are transient lapses in the control of attention focused on your external world that can lead to a shift in focus that is similar to meditation, prayer, or self-vocalization. (Yes, talking to yourself.) As your mind wanders you begin to receive information outside the realm of external consciousness. In a way, your mind automatically defaults to what I call Universal Google, aka Universal Consciousness, to access solutions while awake. These answers may alter your health, love-life, or job, which are often intertwined.

Nearly everyone daydreams on a regular basis. Studies indicate that as many as 96 percent of adults engage in at least one bout of daily daydreaming. This type of dream state is much like a meditative or prayer state.[48]

According to *Psychology Today*, innovative companies give employees time and space to think creatively, that is, daydream. Google offers a 20 percent program, 3M has a 15 percent program, and W. L. Gore & Associates (makers of Gore-Tex), features "dabble time." All three companies credit these programs as the source of their most successful products.[49]

Daydreams have been on the minds of many researchers. William James, the founder of American psychology, studied streams of consciousness for his functionalist theory of the mind. In 1890, he wrote, "When absorbed in the intellectual attention we become so inattentive to outer things as to be 'absent-minded,' or 'abstracted.' He went on to say, "All concentrated meditation is apt to throw us into this state that transient lapses in the control of attention may lead to a shift in attention from the external world to internal meditation." At the University of Leipzig, psychologist Wilhelm Wundt used introspection to understand how the daydreaming mind works.

What does all this research mean? What is the purpose of daydreaming, and how easy is it to daydream? Daydreams enable us to quickly shift into an altered alert state of consciousness through a wandering mind at any time, and in the blink of an eye. All we have to do is shift some of our alert attention from the outside world to our inner world and sail off into a personal Wonderland of Universal Wisdom, or wander along the shore of the Ocean of Gnosis to collect Pearls of Wisdom. In everyday language, mind-wandering in the form of independent thought makes up a daydream.

Daydreaming is also a way for you to remember or reenter an elusive dream. Someone who has trouble remembering their dreams due to medication intake or other physical or psychological trauma can use daydreams as a doorway back into their dream world.

Sleeping is an altered state of alertness, of consciousness, which brings us to lucid dreaming, the state of altered consciousness in which while dreaming you are aware that you are asleep.

Lucid Dreams

Lucid dreams are extremely vivid dreams you have while asleep in which you know you are dreaming. They usually occur just as you drop into a dream state, also referred to as a *hypnogogic state*. The term "lucid" means clear, but lucid dreaming is more than having a clear dream. You must know it is a dream while you are dreaming by being aware of the environment in the dream. Focus on the details in the dream in order to bring them into your waking world for insertion into your dream journal.

With time and practice, you can learn to control the outcome of these dreams to make them emotionally or physically healing dreams. This is particularly true if they are recurring lucid dreams. Changing the ending of a lucid recurring dream may solve a riddle in your life. One listener to my radio program named Linda said she always had trouble falling asleep, never remembered her dreams, but always woke up angry. As she worked on remembering her dreams using the steps outlined in Chapter 30 she remembered why she was angry. Her deceased father kept appearing in her dream, which angered her due to unresolved family issues. The next time her father showed up in her dream she embraced him, told him she forgave and loved him, and the anger stopped. She took control of her lucid dream/nightmare. The new ending was the key to ending her anger and improving her marriage and health.

Nightmares

Nightmares are vividly realistic, disturbing dreams that can jolt you awake from a deep sleep and leave your heart pounding and your body covered in perspiration from fear. They tend to occur when you first fall asleep or in the early morning hours during rapid eye movement (REM) sleep. These are call-to-action dreams that linger after other dreams are forgotten. Despite extreme efforts to forget, who of us cannot remember a frightening dream message? Perhaps the answer is, you are supposed to remember the nightmare because of its importance. Your nightmare may be a gift in disguise. One out of every two adults has nightmares on occasion. And between 2 percent and 8 percent of the adult population is plagued by nightmares.[50] There are many reasons for nightmares.

One is to ensure you remember all the relevant information necessary to solve a problem or work through a situation that could be life-saving. In my case, it was a dream that started off as a spiritually guided lucid dream but shifted into a prophetic healing nightmare when my monk guides dressed as doctors turned into scary circus clowns while holding my mammograms. I got the message, and the details were impossible to forget as described in Part Two. This prophetic lucid nightmare saved my life.

Nightmares may have a significant impact on your quality of life; therefore, it is important to consult a medical professional if you experience them regularly. You can then make changes to reduce their occurrence, which brings us to the next dream category: recurring dreams.

Recurring Dreams

Recurring dreams happen because you did not remember or understand the dream message information the first time, or solve the riddle in the dream. This was seen in many of the multiple dreams of the dreamers in this book. Your inner guidance is using dreams to communicate something important, but you are not "getting it." The majority of recurrent dreams usually appear as nightmares so that you won't dismiss the information. Recurring dreams reflect the presence of an unresolved or persistent conflict in an individual's life. Remember, dreams may speak to us with signs and symbols. If you keep missing the message, your dream environment may shift into a nightmare to get your attention. Recurring dreams appear during tough or emotional times in our lives. Like nightmares, they are also often a call to action.

Healing Dreams

Healing dreams teach you something significant about yourself or someone else and are another call-to-action dream to make a change in your life. They contain emotional or physical information to help heal yourself or a situation and are big, life-changing dreams. If you have had a healing dream in the past, you probably spent weeks, months, even years thinking about its significance. The dream information can be as elusive as an abstract sign or symbol or as concrete as an exact recipe for an ailment delivered by a special person you may or may not know in your waking world. It may be a sentence or conversation heard in the dream given by someone seen or unseen. This person can be an aspect of yourself, a part of your inner guidance such as your Physician-within, an animal, or a spirit guide. Examples of these dreams will be shared in Part Six.

Epic Dreams

Epic dreams are always big in nature. They are also referred to as great dreams, cosmic dreams, or numinous dreams. They are so huge, compelling, and vivid they cannot be ignored. The details of such dreams defy time and space and often remain with you for years, as if you dreamed the dream last night. They possess beauty, contain archetypal symbols and signs, and can be full of conversation by known people or people yet to be known from the future.

They fill you with awe as soon as you awaken by invoking strong emotions that bring about greater awareness of your life from a new perspective. Epic dreams are entertaining and unforgettable information or messages often presented as messages from the "other side." And that brings us to the fantastic dreams that come true: prophetic or precognitive dreams.

Precognitive Dreams

Precognitive dreams come true and can be validated by facts, scientific tests, or life events. Precognitive dreams have many names: prophetic dreams, psychic dreams, primordial dreams, divination dreams, premonition dreams, guided dreams, shamanic dreams, and dreams that come true.

An early inquiry into allegedly prophetic dreams was made by Aristotle in his *On Divination in Sleep.* Belief in precognition has been related to superstition. These dreams are often thought of as superstitions or mere coincidences. The premise of this book is how such "superstitious" coincidences are validated by medical tests.

Precognitive dreams may be remembered as a *déjà vu*, the intense sensation an event or experience currently being experienced has already happened to you in the past, which may have been in the form of a dream. The precognitive dream category is the premise for the research of Dr. Larry Burk in the Breast Cancer Dreams Project, predictive dreams that were later validated by medical reports or life and death.

The chapters in this book written by patients who experienced dreams that came true illuminate the phenomenal ability of humans to see into the future through the next level of dreaming I call the Sacred Dream Doors, which are dream doors within dream doors. Since the book focuses on research into diagnostic and precognitive dreams, three subcategories break down the types of precognitive dreams someone may experience—symbolic, literal, and lucid dreams.

SYMBOLIC: Signs, symbols, and abstract information that may not be understood or realized until the actual event takes place later in the waking world. The remembered dream then takes on new meaning. An example might be a dreamer sees crabs in their house, then finds out they have cancer. Crabs symbolize cancer, and our house symbolizes our body.

LITERAL: A first-person view of the dream in detail, with the message in the dream crystal clear upon awakening. What is heard, sensed, felt, or shown in the dream is understood and comes true in the future. An example might be having someone in a dream tell the dreamer they have cancer and where it is in their body.

LUCID: An alert and focused state of dreaming within the precognitive dream. In his book, *Lucid Dreaming: The Gateway to the Inner Self*,[51] Robert Waggoner, former president of the International Association for the Study of Dreams, wrote about two types of lucid precognitive dreams: *ambient* and *active*. Active lucid precognitive dreams actively engage the dreamer; in an ambient lucid dream, the dreamer passively observes the dream.

In other words, in an active dream the dreamer interacts with the dream rather than watches what is happening in an ambient dream. An example of an ambient dream may be hearing a group of people discussing how a close family friend is ill while knowing you are dreaming. An example of an active lucid dream might be having a dream guide take your hand, place it on your breast, and tell you that you have breast cancer right here. Keep in mind the distinction between the two precognitive dream subcategories as you read the stories in this book.

My *Three Crabs* precognitive dream was an epic, active, lucid, healing recurrent nightmare that came true and was validated by pathology reports, as detailed in Part Two.

How is this possible? One explanation is that we often forget we are not human beings having a spiritual experience on the earth plane; we are spiritual beings housed in a human body having a human experience in life. Our spirit is *in* this terrestrial world but not *of* this world. Therefore, I believe we are partially **e**xtra-**t**errestrial (ET). Our dreams are our inner-ET phoning home for information or helping us deal with human challenges. What is amazing is that someone on the "other side" always answers the phone. Categorizing and defining your dreams will help you remember the answers to your inner-ET's questions and the answers you receive.

Waking Dreams

Waking dreams often involve what is described as a hallucinatory feeling that occurs in the transitional state between wakefulness and sleep, defined as *hypnogogic*, the threshold of consciousness. Waking dreams often include lucid dream thoughts, lucid dream voices, lucid dreaming, a feeling of falling that can result in a sudden physical jerk, and occasionally a sense of having hallucinations and "sleep paralysis" in which the dreamer is unable to move.

Dream journaling can help you learn to distinguish between the different types of dreams and their messages. Now that you know the eight basic dreams, you are ready to immerse yourself in the stories of the dream team from the Breast Cancer Dream Project in Part Two and to start working on your own dream skills in Part Four.

PART TWO

True Stories of the Breast Cancer Research Team

I would not deny the possibility of parallel dreams,
i.e., dreams whose meaning coincides with or supports
the conscious attitude, but in my experience,
at least, these are rather rare.
— CARL JUNG, *CW 12, Para 48*

These are the personal stories and dreams of the participants in Dr. Larry Burk's Breast Cancer Dreams Project. Watch for the universal dream symbols, signs, and play on words in their amazing dreams, which will be explained in Kat's interpretation at the end of each dream and Dr. Burk's commentary at the end of each dream story, which focuses on the dreams from a more medical point of view.

Many of these women had a series of guided dreams, consisting of multiple dreams that began with a diagnostic dream and continued with healing dreams for guidance and life. Although these series of dreams might be considered recurrent in nature by some dream experts, they often appeared as steps, or dream doors within doors, opening to the next dream level of life saving.

Introduction

Suzanne Maria De Gregorio,
Triple Positive Breast Cancer Survivor

With regard to prognosis, therefore, dreams are often in a
much more favorable position than consciousness.
— CARL JUNG, *CW 8, Para 493*

I don't write this introduction to our stories to say, "Look at us. We have this superpower," because we don't. We have what everyone else has—dreams. I'd rather take a nap, and I would not expect it to interest anyone else, either. However, if we are right, that heeding our warning dreams of illness saved our lives, this may have relevance beyond our own experiences.

Sharing our stories might inspire others to pay closer attention to their own health-related dreams. It could encourage doctors to listen carefully when such cases present, as did Wanda Burch's surgeon. The reality is, we need more tools for breast cancer screening. Might dreams be one we can add to our health toolbox?

Can people be trained to tune in to their bodies to detect health problems early, as we in the study appear to have done spontaneously? That potentially life-saving question is worth asking, and research is the most logical place to start.

This book is a call for such studies, and I'm grateful to Dr. Burk for taking the pioneering first steps in that direction. My website, *Moonbeams and Eco-Dreams,* was never meant to be about me. It is the backbone of the following interviewed dream stories from the co-participants in Dr. Larry Burk's study of breast cancer warning dreams published in the May/June 2015 issue of *Explore: The Journal of Science and Healing.*

Kat's Two Cents

Many of the following dream stories describe life as **BC** (**B**efore **C**ancer) and **AD** (**A**fter **D**iagnosis). Cancer is such a life-changing experience it has the potential to divide survivors lives into two segments, much like the Bible—BC and AD.

6

"It's Your Time to Get Cancer!"

Suzanne Maria De Gregorio

"No matter how many lumps you've had checked out
that turned out to be cysts, never assume.
Let the doctors tell you what is and is not cancer."

My body screamed warnings at me during the year leading up to my diagnosis. In retrospect, I see just how stark they were. But I put them in the back of my mind at the time because they seemed so bizarre. I think you will agree.

How My Body Knew Before I Did

During the summer of 2013, a sentence kept awakening me in the middle of the night: *It's time for you to get cancer.*

I ignored the thought because it pissed me off. Perhaps my brain was just screwing with me, like a recurrent nightmare or something. By day, I mocked these terrifying suggestions ("Gee, I forgot I made that cancer-getting appointment. How inconvenient"); by night, I worried what cruel claim my subconscious would submit next for my consideration. But mostly, life went on as normal; that is, until my next routine breast screening that winter.

An Archetype from Beyond

A local woman named Cheryl had died of cancer a few years earlier. She was a friend of a friend. About five months before receiving my breast cancer diagnosis, I could not stop thinking about Cheryl, which was strange since I didn't know her and we had never met. It was almost like something about her was trying to break through my consciousness and get my attention.

I told our mutual friend this at church one day, and we sought to figure out what it could mean. I am not implying that the spirit of a stranger was trying to give me a dire warning from beyond. I just think my body was using Cheryl as an archetype to warn me that I too had cancer, but I did not pick up on it. Both of my parents had had cancer, so it would be normal for me

54

to think about them. This had to be a person I had no reason whatsoever to think about that intently. That is why my psyche chose to focus on Cheryl just before my mammogram.

My Life Kept Flashing Before Me

In the fall of 2013, my life started flashing before me. Every few hours I would get flashes of memories from childhood that I had completely forgotten, followed by stuff from my teen years, then something from adulthood. It was always poignant, different each time; like playing with a beloved toy, my first crush, seeing my husband for the first time, watching my son take his first steps. Though much got packed into the memories, they were over in a flash, until the next one. This had never happened to me before, and it was jarring. I said to my husband, "My God, it is like what they say happens when you're dying." It has not happened again since I was diagnosed. Again, I think my body was trying to get my attention.

When my previous mammogram had been read as normal, the radiologist casually mentioned that I have dense breasts. Having more fibrous than fatty breast tissue, mammograms sometimes miss malignancies in women with this condition.

I Became One of Them

Haunted by those dreams, but under no medical suspicion of cancer, I requested an MRI that year since that technology detects abnormalities better through dense tissue than mammography. Surely it couldn't hurt with my history of cysts, plus my mother had in situ breast cancer at the age of 49. An abundance of caution, I assured myself. That is all.

When medical intuition first strikes, you mentally banter back and forth like that. Though motivated by the information, there is also doubt. It's human nature to want to believe we are just fine, that our health is not in jeopardy.

The Lady Who Diagnosed Me
with Breast Cancer in a Dream

Then another ominous dream invaded my sleep. Between getting scanned and receiving the results, I dreamed:

> A woman in a white lab coat told me I had breast cancer. She said to me,
> "You have stage 3 breast cancer."

The dream could not be rationalized away. It was not general fear phrases pushing through the night like before. The symbolism here was clear; an actual medical person was telling me I had cancer. I can still see that woman's face, her short curly hair. I would recognize her on the street to this day.

"This thing will come back positive," I told my husband. "I have breast cancer."

One week and a biopsy later, her words were confirmed by my real-life doctor, though the stage was unknown. During lumpectomy, the surgeon would stain lymph nodes near the breast. If cells light up in any regional nodes that means the cancer has spread and all affected nodes must go immediately. Even if no nodes are positive the surgeon still sacrifices one to be sure. When the dissected sample returns clear of cancer cells, depending on tumor size, it could mean stage 1 or less. My tumor was 1.8 centimeters, small enough for stage 1, should my nodes look normal.

My cancer was stage 1, but in the dream, she said stage 3. If the dream was correct about my having cancer did that also mean it was right about stage 3? Long-term survival prospects for stage 3 breast cancer patients, I understood, can be somewhat low. They were about to cut off half my breast, and I could almost care less. If I woke up from surgery with a death sentence, would it really matter if I'm lopsided?

"Wake up. It is time to wake up." I heard her voice but couldn't see. There were people groaning in pain around me, but I couldn't see them either.

"How many did they take from me?" I pleaded. "How many?"

"One lymph node," said the voice in the room.

"Oh, thank God. I'm going to live." I whispered, beginning to stir, then joined the a chorus of groans around me.

My final pathology diagnosis was stage 1 HER2 (+3) breast cancer that previous mammograms had missed. At 43 years of age, I was six years younger than my mother when she was diagnosed with breast cancer. Mine was a very aggressive tumor that had not yet spread. Would a mammogram alone have missed it again, destining me for diagnosis at a later, less treatable stage? Quite possibly.

Some of you may be thinking: *Stage 1? Good for you! Don't you get to dodge chemo, just do radiation, and take that estrogen pill?* That is what I used to think. But not so fast. Some of us do require chemo. I had triple positive HER2 invasive ductal carcinoma. HER2 malignancies are so aggressive that without chemo and Herceptin, 40 percent of stage 1's are dead within five years. Stray cells can sometimes get into the bloodstream without affecting the lymph nodes. Chemo and Herceptin increase the five-year survival rate to 85 percent by zapping those wayward cells before they can form metastatic tumors.

Avoiding chemo was never a realistic option for me, but that didn't stop me from convincing myself it could be. The emotional push-pulls of dueling percentages tore at my being, day and night; yet there, in the background, the dream doctor's words still worked on me. *You have stage 3 breast cancer.*

But, I did not have stage 3. My clear lymph nodes said so! Was the dream suggesting that I'm at risk for another cancer in the future? Or was it warning me that this cancer was more serious than it seemed? I considered the symbolism of stage 3: serious but treatable. Stray cells, then? Ugh! I needed an undeniable answer.

"Don't leave me alone with him!" my husband said after our daily go-round about chemo. He was referring to our 11-year-old special-needs son, Alex. (The story of healing his seizures with medical cannabis guided by my dreams will be told later in Chapter 47.)

That hit me square in the maternal instinct. I had been thinking only in terms of myself: my body, my health, my choice. But it was not only my choice, nor should it be. When we are committed to others, when they depend on us, we must consider them. My husband wasn't comforted by the greater likelihood my surgeon had already cured me. He worried about the 40 percent chance that without further treatment I'd be dead in five years. He didn't want to lose his wife or our son to lose his mother. Even if I ultimately died, I needed to know I had done all I could do to live for them. I took the chemo.

My Precognitive Dream Came True

Before beginning treatment, I met with a local cancer counselor. A volunteer led me into a room and asked me to wait there. When the counselor walked in, my eyes went straight to her short curly hair, then to her facial features. I would know this woman anywhere. It was the lady who diagnosed me with cancer in my dream! She told me she was a nurse and a breast cancer survivor. That explains the lab coat in the dream. She also said all her axillary nodes were removed during treatment, so that's what, at least stage 3? Was that confirmation of my chemo decision? Who knows? I knew nothing anymore.

I learned to dialogue with my sleeping psyche to heal my body during chemotherapy. And there is an upside. No longer running in multiple directions at once, I am actually more focused and productive than ever. I had always been intense about social justice, often over-committed. It's like I tried to regulate my anxiety about the state of the world by working enough for five citizens. There were my full-time job and the 30-plus hours of unpaid work on my various causes.

No longer able to do this, physically or mentally, I finally understand that I never really could. Before cancer I shot arrows in many directions, hoping to hit the mark somewhere. Knowing my limits, and no longer so spread out, I manage a busy food pantry, cook healthy food from scratch, and raise my high-needs child. These days I offer one citizen's contribution to the world, and it is enough.

I believe our subconscious minds actually dialogue with us, but we don't always notice. The topics of these conversations are induced by our most intense desires. For me, one of these has always been health. Few matters occupy my mental bandwidth quite like the chase for well-being. For years, I'd been setting intentions to receive healing information for myself and my son, Alex. Expecting answers, I paid attention. For Alex, those answers appeared gradually, like bread crumbs to be followed; for me, like a thud in the night.

The Black Owl Messenger

A year before my diagnosis I was treated for a phobia by my friend, hypnotherapist Rebecca Geracitano. My subconscious went deep during this session, and some mechanism was apparently released. Soon, precognitive dreams began tumbling out of me, and you know the rest. Neither of us saw that coming. After my diagnosis, we did another session. We wanted to identify how my mind might assist in the healing process. Again, neither of us could have predicted what happened next. After the induction, an image of a large black owl appeared in front of me, seeming almost nose to nose with me. Not mentioning this to Rebecca, I was terrified—the owl can be a symbolic messenger of death. For some reason, I began referring to myself in the third person, as if speaking of someone else.

"She hasn't decided yet if she will live," said whatever that was.

"What do you mean?" asked Becky.

"She's exhausted. Years of watching her son suffer, helpless to make it better. On some level, she's done. She feels like she's failed. But, there is still time. If she decides to, she will live; if not, she will go."

I am ashamed to tell you this, but at that moment I paused and wondered if I could live this life anymore. I had been traumatized, and there was never time to fully feel that. But there in that quiet office, in the presence of a trusted friend, I owned my anguish and chose life.

"She has decided to live, and she will be a voice." The black owl appeared again, this time at a distance, eyeing me from a perch.

A voice? For breast cancer? Seriously? I was still fighting for my son's access to medical cannabis for his epilepsy, being a voice there. When all that was over I would get to be done with being a voice, or so I thought.

But I couldn't shake what had happened to us. Why did we dream of having cancer before actually being diagnosed? And if we are right, that heeding the warning dreams saved our lives, the outcomes may have relevance beyond our own experiences. If sharing my story might encourage others to pay closer attention to health-related signals suggested in their sleep, then I must be a voice.

Today I am more alive than ever. Though distressing, I never refer to my precognitive cancer dreams as nightmares. Not anymore. They were gifts from my psyche. Had their warning not been heeded, by now I might be planning my end of life care instead of my next vacation. I don't dream because I live, but rather, as Wanda Burch says, "I live because I dream."

Being a Part of Dr. Larry Burk's Dream Study

More shocking than being diagnosed with cancer in a dream was learning that I was in good company, that diagnostic and precognitive dreaming is actually *a thing*.

KAT'S DREAM INTERPRETATION

If these were my dreams, I would have understood them much as Suzanne did because she is an avid Diagnostic and Precognitive Dreamer. Like some of the other dreamers in the study, she heard voice messages telling her she had cancer but also had a literal and symbolic dream. The dream in which the medical person walked up to her in the dream and told her she had cancer was validated by pathology reports. Suzanne can ride the Time Continuum in her dreams of which Albert Einstein often spoke. In the dream world, there is no past or future, just the Big Now. The problem was determining which dream was just entertaining and which was a life-saving precognitive dream showing the future.

Suzanne understood that using the dead friend of a friend as an archetype of death while you watch your life pass before you is a waking daydream, and an important message that does not need symbolic interpretation—it needs to be listened to. If this were my dream, like Suzanne, I would believe it was meant to turn on a mental light bulb. Suzanne's dreams are also full of a play on words rather than symbols. Her dream stating she had stage 3 cancer may have been the HER2 +3. If *an owl* visited my dream, it would make my night and may mean the intuitive part of me is calling to Universal Wisdom. An owl sees what is happening in the dark unconscious areas of your soul and brings you wisdom and insight. Think, Wise Old Owl. Just as an owl can turn its head all the way around to create the circle of life, it can observe all things from within the circle. To have an owl visit your dream may symbolize your expanded awareness in the mystical world beyond the veil of night.

DR. BURK'S COMMENTARY

Suzanne's HER2 diagnosis on the pathology report refers to human epidermal growth factor receptor 2, which means that a gene mutation results in overproduction of this protein, leading to the more rapid growth of the breast cancer. It does make for a scarier prognosis, but having a precognitive dream that came true about the woman in the white coat was definitely a confidence builder that she was on the right track. I suspect it also helped her in processing the owl imagery and making the positive decision to live. Thus far, it seems that the ability to dream the diagnosis of breast cancer among the study group has been a good predictor of successful healing, although more research will be needed to verify that claim.

7

Our Bleeding Breasts?
A Mother-Daughter Dream Team

Amparo Trujillo and Rocio Aguirre

*"I believe that we need to become acquainted with different ways of
knowing and being in the world, and dreams are a great way to do it.
Make of your dreams a valuable resource of inner wisdom."*
— ROCIO AGUIRRE, *Dreamer*

Amparo does not speak English, so her daughter Rocio acts as a translator
for this chapter. Rocio's own dreams leading up to her mother's diagnosis
are featured at the end.

Bleeding Breasts Dream

I am in my apartment, lying down on my bed, when I notice a lot of blood
coming out of both of my breasts, as if they were hurt. My breasts are naked,
and blood is running down my skin. I feel anguish, concern, and so terrified the
dream awakes me.

My name is Rocio, and this is my mother, Amparo's, dream several months before
her June 1, 2012, breast cancer diagnosis. Although she had received information
from dreams much of her life, Mom did not immediately connect this one to
her own health. She associated it with mine. A cyst had recently been found in
my breast. She wondered if the dream was telling us something about the cyst.

I knew otherwise. You see, I had been having dreams of my own for some
time, which caused me to be concerned about my mother.

My mom, Amparo Trujillo, has lived in Ibague, Colombia, almost all her life.
My father's death forced her into unfamiliar territory. Since Dad made all the
major decisions and was her financial support, not only did Mom lose her life
partner but she also suddenly had to figure out those responsibilities on her
own. Mom moved from the home she shared with her husband for about 33
years into an apartment and was learning to live independently. Then cancer
struck. This is her story about a dream that saved her life.

My Dream Said I Had Cancer

My name is Amparo, and I have two daughters who live in different cities. One of them is translating this chapter for me, and she is also an avid dreamer. As a retired woman, I spend most of my time doing exercises, reading, participating in social and family events, and activities that nurture me physically, mentally, and spiritually. Singing is one of my loves. Before my retirement, I was a professional singer and continued performing for fun from time to time at social or family events.

At the time my dream told me of my breast cancer, I was still grieving. Two years earlier my husband had died in an accident, which was very shocking for everyone. Or it was for me. I didn't realize my daughter was dreaming of his accident.

While I was still very affected by this crisis, and not fully recovered from my grief, my daughters moved me from my home of 33 years to a smaller but more comfortable apartment. At the same time, learning how to be more independent and making my own decisions was a full-time job. This was the beginning of an entirely new stage in my life, in more ways than one.

As an avid dreamer, I had always received information through dreams, but this particular unexpected dream frightened me. It was also my first dream about something seriously affecting my health. Once awakened, the same feelings continue to flow over me. I had a hunch my oldest daughter Rocio (who is translating this for me) could be in danger, because the doctors had discovered a cyst in her breast. I thought the dream was a warning for her. I never imagined this was about myself.

I told my daughter Rocio about my dream, and she encouraged me to go see the doctor as soon as possible. She had a hunch the dream was not about her. However, I did not do the screening immediately, but waited and went to the doctor a couple of months later.

My Dream Validation

The outcome of my testing was cancer in my left breast that could be treated with a mastectomy alone and a drug for five years to prevent further cancer. The dream had been about me after all.

Generally, doctors are skeptics concerning warning or precognitive dreams, so I did not tell my physician or the medical staff about the dream. However, my dream, and the subsequent actions taken due to the dream, saved my life because the cancer was discovered in time. I did not need aggressive radiation or chemotherapy treatments; only a mastectomy.

Dr. Larry Burk's Dream Study

I became included in Dr. Larry Burk's study when my daughter, Rocio, was participating in the PsiberDreaming Conference organized by the IASD (International Association for the Study of Dreams) in September/October 2013. Dr. Burk was a presenter about diagnostic dream topics and asked for volunteers for his research on warning dreams and breast cancer. Rocio told me about it, and I was interested in talking about my story.

If I had anything else to share with you about my experience with dreams that can come true and save lives, it is this: make your dreams a valuable resource of inner wisdom. So write them down, pay attention to them, and learn to interpret the symbols that come through them. They are an extraordinary way to guide you in all areas of your life!

KAT'S INTERPRETATION

If this were my dream I would take it as literally as Amparo did, making it a literal diagnostic dream that left no doubt about the message; her breasts were bleeding and unhealthy. In a figurative sense, her broken heart was bleeding, too, possibly making this dream a duality; two messages in one dream. With her family's history of breast cysts, it might be normal to imagine the dream is meant for another family member. However, she saw herself in the dream. This is an example of an active dreaming, where the dreamer actively participates, as it also shows her future mastectomy. Fortunately, her daughter convinced her to see a doctor, which saved her life. The dream was diagnostic, because it was validated by a pathology report. Often, we can dream for ourselves, and in the process even share dreams about others, making them another kind of duality; like dreaming with and for others, as shared in Part Eight.

DR. BURK'S COMMENTARY

Breast cancer may be preceded by a significant emotional trauma prior to diagnosis as in Amparo's case. The death of her husband represented a major blow to the heart chakra and also the fire element in the Chinese five-element system. The fire element controls the blood vessels related to hemorrhage and nourishes the earth element, which is associated with the stomach meridian that runs through the breasts. The imbalance in the earth element results in a tendency to nurture others instead of yourself. Fire also controls the metal element, which is associated with the emotion of grief.

Rocio's Dreams

I have been working in the corporate world within the learning industry for more than 20 years. A few years ago, I felt a strong calling to serve others and embarked on a journey of self-discovery and healing, which led me to pursue a new career that brought more meaning to my life.

A Major Change in My Life

This was a significant shift for me because I had always been very left-brained and a linear thinker, so connecting with my spiritual right-brain intuition in the waking state was difficult. It started with dreams when my conscious mind could not filter the information. As I learned to trust, I could get tremendous support from my inner guidance. It is my belief that we need to become acquainted with different ways of knowing and being in the world. Dreams are a great way to start. We need an approach to embracing diversity and integrative thinking that encourages us to change our fragmented worldview for a wider perspective. We are part of a bigger, more interrelated whole.

Let us return to my dreams and my mom.

My dreams started more than a year before Mom was diagnosed with cancer. The same thing happened with my father's death. My dreams about his death began more than a year before he had the accident.

The Dreams I Had About My Mother and Her Breast Cancer

The dreams began February 16, 2011:

Is Mom Sick?

I'm in an unknown place with many people. Some people are sitting while others are lying on the floor. Somebody is sick. I think it is my mom. I see hospital stuff, devices. Someone is giving orders.

Five Days Later: Exposed Breast

While standing in line at a hotel counter, I see my friend Adri next to me. She is wearing a black transparent short dress. Suddenly, I realize I'm staring at her breast. When she notices it, I feel embarrassed and try to explain, "I see you didn't put on a bra, and everything is exposed."

September 1, 2011: The Bag with Medical Stuff

I'm in a room in a house with several rooms. My Auntie Orlanda is with me and hands me a bag filled with medical stuff, including shots and rubber bands.

It is sent by my cousin, who is a doctor. Although I don't need it now, it should be kept for future use. During the same night, I had another dream—someone very close to me is sick, but I can't remember who she is.

Thirteen Days Later: The Intubation

I am in a house after visiting the hospital. I feel something on my back and begin to pull a long and thin tube out of my back. I'm scared! (What's that?)
I notice many more tubes coming out of my body. I am intubated... for oxygen?
My parents are with me. Should the health insurance be called to ask them to remove those tubes from my body? Would it be painful, I wonder?
My doctor cousin is by my side, but she cannot do it, so I go to a room where the procedure can be done. I ring a bell, and a doctor's assistant appears to escort me to a little room to change my clothes. Two doctors are relaxing on a table.

All this reminds me of the drainage tubes Mom had after her mastectomy in August 2012. Two medical specialists took care of the surgery: an oncologist and a plastic surgeon.

Oct 11, 2011: The Stain of Blood

There is a blood stain on a woman's body. It seems to be coming out of her breast.

There was a time I thought dreams had little significance to offer concerning our health. But that changed after my father was tragically killed in a bike accident. I'd been dreaming of his death a year and a half before it happened, but never thought at the time these were precognitive dreams until I opened my dream journal afterward and saw these stark warnings in ominous detail. It is amazing what my subconscious is capable of knowing.

More Rocio Dreams

In the first dream, I'm consoling my mother and sister, saying, "Dad is dead, but he's okay, and we'll be fine, too." The next dream has me at the scene of a bike accident. The victim is a man I do not recognize. We are there alone in the dark, and I yell into the night for someone to help me because this man is dying. Coincidentally, this is how my father died later, alone, on a dark road at night. The final dream has me again with my mother and my sister, but this one is a bit more symbolic. Mom is passing me three black blouses. The symbolism is clear: black is the universal color for mourning.

Despite my pressure, at first, Mom refused to go to the doctor. No surprise there. Fearing bad news, Mom always avoided doctor visits as much as possible. But eventually doubt crept in. What if the dream had been a warning about *her* health? Not to mention, I had all those dreams suggesting a problem. And, why was she suddenly seeing breast cancer everywhere: on television, awareness events, fund-raisers? Could these be omens?

Now, thank goodness, Mom was more afraid of *not* seeing a doctor. She was diagnosed with cancer in her left breast, detected early enough to avoid chemotherapy and radiation. Had my mother ignored our warnings dreams and continued her lifelong pattern of dodging doctor visits she may not have been so fortunate.

Like the other women in Dr. Burk's study, cancer jolted Mom's mind into sharp focus as she reviewed her life thus far. Had she enjoyed it to its fullest? Did she spend too much time worrying about unimportant things? And, if she survived, how did she want to spend her remaining years? The dream suggested the existence of an inner guidance system she could access along the way, which gave her confidence.

These days, Mom seems to enjoy herself more. She favors activities that nurture her physically, mentally, and spiritually, such as singing. All her soul searching about worry has my mother less apprehensive about the details of life. Running from one activity to the next is no longer her way. Mom's pace is slower now—with the flow, no longer ahead of it.

As for me, Rocio, I too learned something from these tragic and mysterious episodes, which consumed my family.

Before my father's fatal accident and my mother's cancer, I was unaware that my dreams could predict future events, so naturally, my mind didn't connect those three dreams to Dad. But once understood, vital information can indeed come to us through sleep. My intuition radar was on high alert when bloody breast dreams began haunting Mom and me. She was getting to the doctor one way or another. I'd make sure of it.

Now I work as a life coach, encouraging others to learn their unique dream language. Not all dreams lay out concerns in literal detail. There is often symbolism to decode, sometimes as a mix of literal and symbolic composites across time, as with my dreams concerning Mom and Dad. We can track this in dream journals to pinpoint where to focus our attention.

Today, I am a certified professional coach with an M.A. in Transpersonal Psychology, and have studied a variety of healing modalities, such as mindfulness, art therapy, EFT, and dreamwork.

KAT'S INTERPRETATION

These dreams are an example of dreaming for others, also seen in the next dream story with Paulette Wyssbrod-Goltz, and is a dream-subject explained in depth in Part Eight of the book. If these were my dreams, I would define them as precognitive nightmares, with recurrent messages that were active, symbolic and literal. The dreams were validated by pathology reports and contained signs and symbols understood in the waking world, such as breasts, blood, hospitals, doctors, and tubes coming out of the dreamer's chest and back. The dreams were literal because they were viewed in the first person, and the message in the dream was clear upon awakening.

DR. BURK'S COMMENTARY

My IASD PsiberDreaming presentation was the beginning of my launch of the Breast Cancer Dreams Project, and I was pleased when Rocio offered her mother's story. Due to the language barrier, I didn't fully appreciate the extent of the dreaming connection between Rocio and Amparo until after the interview by Suzanne, so I am grateful for those details. With the genetic tendency of breast cancer often being shared by mother and daughter, it is also no surprise that other breast cancer dreamers have reported that this connection extends beyond death in the dreamworld, where deceased mothers and grandmothers appear as guides from the other side.

8

"Your Mother Has Cancer."
Another Mother-Daughter Dream Team

Paulette Wyssbrod-Goltz

*"If you have a dream that warns you about a health condition, push it
until someone listens to you, regardless of their response."*

*Your mother has cancer, she has three months to live, and you have a tumor in
your right breast.* "What?!" I turned on my bedside lamp, scanned the room
to see if anyone was there, then looked at the clock. It was just after 2 a.m. The
next day I told my sister about the dream.

A few weeks later my mother was diagnosed with cervical cancer and given
three months to live. She made it to six.

When my breast cancer dreams began, I was single, had just moved back
to Houston, Texas, from southern California, and was working as a manager
for a large multi-family housing company. It was a high-stress job because it
was a rather new concept called LIHTC, the acronym for Low-Income Housing
Tax Credit pronounced "lie-tech," a dollar-for-dollar tax credit in the U.S. for
affordable housing investments, also known as Section 42 credits.

There was so much more to the job than traditional management. I called
it working for corporate America, and the money was good. Basically, it was a
time in my life when everything was going my way, including the freedom to do
whatever I wanted with friends, family, and so on. Dreams about health issues
were not common for me, and this dream surprised me. I have always had message dreams, but never about health.

Do I Have Cancer, Too?

Since the dream was correct about my mother having cervical cancer, did
it also mean there was a tumor in my right breast? I had to know. Both my
regular doctor and my oncologist did not respond to my dream. I saw the
same oncologist my mother had had, and I told her about the dream. She was
a feisty, old doctor who listened but said nothing. However, I did go early for
another screening after the dream. All of my mammograms for the next few
years were *supposedly* okay. Never one to miss those annual screenings since my

two sisters and paternal grandfather all had breast cancer, I dutifully continued my commitment and felt relieved each time the mammograms returned clear.

Four years after the dream, things began to change. A screening report received by mail stated I had breast calcifications, but no immediate follow up was suggested. It turns out those initially ignored calcifications were malignant. But since no further investigation was recommended by a doctor, it did not occur to me to request one. A biopsy and diagnosis a year earlier may have spared me much of what came next.

I Found My Cancer While Getting Dressed One Morning

The following year a flakey orange peel-looking patch, the size of a silver dollar, appeared on my right breast. The minute I saw it, I knew what it was and returned to the center that had always done my screenings. I was livid when the practitioner refused to investigate my new orange peel symptom beyond mammography. My primary doctor palpated the area, declared nothing amiss, but recommended a mammogram anyhow.

"Look, you need to take a more serious look at this!"

"No," replied the female doctor. "Let's just do the mammogram."

"No. No. NO! We are not doing that. Last year, you sent a letter saying I had calcifications, recommended no follow up, and now I have this orange thing on my boob!" I fumed, storming out of her office.

Luckily a doctor in Houston was willing to see me right away.

"Oh my God!" she exclaimed, examining the flakey orange silver dollar on my breast.

"I need to get another mammogram," I told her. "I know what this is, and don't care what the last mammogram said."

She performed a mammogram in which the technicians put sticky things around the area of the orange peel skin. I waited for the results. Within an hour they sent me in for an ultrasound and biopsy. I knew I had breast cancer. Three days later, it was confirmed by a pathology report. The breast cancer in my right breast would require an aggressive treatment plan.

It turns out those initially ignored calcifications were malignant. I was eventually diagnosed with stage 2 estrogen-positive breast cancer in three lymph nodes. It turned out the tumor had probably been growing in me for about five years. My dream was in the late summer of 1998, and the diagnosis was November 2003, five years later. I had taken all the right actions by following through with yearly mammograms and doing breast exams, but none of that helped in finding the cancer. My dream did.

My cancer was missed the first time, so I could not implicitly trust any doctor's recommendations, especially since they involved poisoning me. Why must I take chemo, the Red Devil also known as Adriamycin, when just a few years earlier my same cancer was treatable with only Tamoxifen? And why wasn't there some other way to rid my body of stray cells short of pumping it with toxins? My inner tug-of-war caused much wrangling between us, but this physician had deep roots in my family. She was my mother's oncologist who later planned to treat my father's pancreatic cancer. So I chose to trust her and take the poisons, to my regret.

Before chemo I had a double radical mastectomy, the easiest decision I had to make in this entire process, given my substantial family history of breast cancer. Plus, I was never really comfortable with "those breasts" anyhow.

By 8th grade I was a 38C and wearing baggy sweatshirts to cover them up, beginning a lifelong project to conceal those girls from unwanted male attention. I looked forward to brand new reconstructed B cups that stood at attention.

My mastectomy surgery was 16 hours long, followed by immediate reconstruction with implants. But one of the newbies developed an infection, prompting its removal. We decided on skin graft reconstruction a year after chemo instead of saline. But alas, that was not to be either.

Once the surgeon started talking about taking skin from my back for the rebuilding process, I said, "No! I'm not doing this. I'm done having breasts." I have no regrets about the mastectomy or foregoing reconstruction. It's okay. Really! I was never comfortable with those things anyhow, remember?

The Rest of My Treatment Plan, However, Is Another Story

My cocktail of necessity, or so I was told, was Adriamycin (the Red Devil) and Taxol. The Taxol brought on Bell's palsy nerve damage, which caused the right side of my face and eye to droop.

Worse still was the aromatase inhibitor I had to take for five years to block estrogen from feeding stray cancer cells. After three months on the drug, my hands were swollen to the size of baseball gloves and the joints throughout my body were stiff. I knew it was the drug.

"My other patients aren't having this problem," said my family oncologist.

"I don't care about your other patients. I care that my hands are baseball gloves!"

The drug was stopped, but the damage was done. My joints locked, which made it hard to move. I took long-term disability.

Before cancer my life was satisfying. I worked for a large real estate corporation, managing a multi-million-dollar enterprise and a staff of 20. The money was good. I had just bought a condo. My children were grown, leaving plenty of time to pursue my interests which included classes toward the psychology degree I had always wanted and attending metaphysical seminars with friends. Then a 2 a.m. dream one morning launched me toward a whole new reality.

Dr. Larry Burk's Dream Study

Dr. Larry Burk's dream study caught my attention when I saw it on Dr. Christiane Northrup's Facebook page. It was about being told you have breast cancer in a dream. If my dream had been taken seriously and used for early detection of breast cancer by the medical staff, my treatment and life would be very different now.

Family Deaths

Like my peers in Dr. Burk's study, I'm amazed by how I surf life's challenges differently now compared with before cancer. In 2008, my brother committed suicide. Before my illness, I would have lost control. I still don't like that it happened, and do not advocate suicide as a solution for anyone, but I understand why he did it. Some people get through life's challenges, and for whatever reasons, some do not. And when my sister died of brain cancer in 2015, I navigated that wave as well, and still do. Some people survive cancer, and for whatever reasons, some do not. We are simply approaching that age where some of us will start dying. My loved ones died, and if they did it, when my time comes I can die, too. Before cancer, I would have been sacked by grief's undertow, but after cancer, it's all a process to me now.

In Conclusion: Self-Advocate

However, acceptance of things we can't change does not mean we shouldn't fight like hell for what we know. What if I'd acquiesced to that first doctor's office where they only wanted to do a mammogram, the same office that failed to follow up on those calcifications, despite my substantial family history of breast cancer?

If I hadn't pushed for a biopsy against their judgment, my cancer would have been caught at a later stage, and I might not be here to write this. Doctors know many things, but they don't know everything. At your fingertips online, you have access to many of the same studies as physicians do, but you need their help interpreting them.

Read. Research. Ask Questions.

For instance, since my paternal grandfather and two sisters had breast cancer, why did nobody ever suggest an occasional MRI, since mammography can miss tumors in some women?

So, if you think you have a problem with a doctor, get a new one. It could save your life. My career, as I knew it, is now over. No longer able to work and settling into a slower-paced life, I returned to school and finished my BS degree in Psychology. Requiring two more classes to graduate, I decided to take creative writing I and II. Writing has always been a passion. Now, there was more time to work on my two young adult fiction books for a series contracted to a publisher. Although cancer has cost me much, I love being able to write. Would I have had time to explore this creativity if I had remained in the workforce? I doubt it.

Fourteen years later I'm still here, still living fully, and despite it all, cancer free. I am a writer/author, now living in a small town on the Texas coast. As a freelance writer for three online platforms, my pen name is used to self-publish on Amazon. If you have a dream that warns you about a health condition, push it until someone listens to you, regardless of their response.

KAT'S INTERPRETATION

Paulette's dream is similar to Suzanne's and Rocio's, because like Suzanne, she heard a voice, and like Rocio, it was also about her mother. Paulette not only dreamed for herself but also for another person, as seen later in Part Eight of this book. If this were my dream, I would consider it auditory in nature, making it a literal precognitive dream because it foretold cancer five years before it began to grow, and was discovered and validated by pathology reports five years later.

This dreamer did not interact with the dream. This is one dream for two people that wakes Paulette at 2 a.m. *The number 2* is a reinforced symbolism for balance, duality, and the second chakra, dealing with self, which is carried over into the waking world. If this were my dream, I would define it as an inactive auditory precognitive and diagnostic dream. The dream came true and was validated by pathology reports.

DR. BURK'S COMMENTARY

The delay between Paulette's dream and her diagnosis was much longer than most of the other women in the study, although there was another woman with a nine-year delay. The fact that she didn't ignore the dream due to its accurate diagnosis of her mother, and actively sought out screening year after year, reminds us that what is considered early detection through mammography may not be as soon as we would like it to be.

Mammography is not a perfect test, and interpretation of the significance of calcifications requires considerable skill. In her case, a more sensitive MRI scan might have been more useful, based on the risk factors in her family history. Perhaps someday, with more research documentation, having a warning dream will be added to the list of risk factors.

9

"I Had a Dream."

Diane Long

Sooner or later, a period of chaos mushrooms into everyone's life.
It could be a natural disaster, illness, old age, or loss of a loved one.
Yet it is with this chaos... a new meaning could awaken within us,
which will require an introspective path of thinking.
This new perception of thought can open your heart to everything
that is connected to this element of being human."

My home-based floral studio specializes in weddings and, often, matters of the heart. In late January 2011, a client called and asked for flowers to be sent to a friend.

"Could you design a floral arrangement, something with more scent, like lavender or gardenias?" my client asked. "I want the flowers sent to a sister-in-law in hospice care."

She had found my business website online and was struck by my physical resemblance to her ailing friend. "You look so much like her. She always smiled and loved life but has simply lost her battle to cancer."

A Few Nights Later I Had a Dream.

I was having lunch with my cousin and telling her I had the big C: cancer. However, we were laughing, giggling, and telling funny stories. So when I woke up, it was not with dread but a fleeting thought of my last week's client and the flowers for her friend.

A couple days later I came down with 24-hour flu-like symptoms, with a fever and really sore muscles. I thought I had played too much tennis the day before. The following day, a deep pain developed in my left breast with a red dot. Two days later the dot grew to the size of a half-dollar.

The enlarging mark and penetrating pain led me to suspect inflammatory breast cancer. As in Kat's story, convincing doctors to take my cancer concerns seriously would be an emotional tug-of-war.

An appointment was made with my medical group HMO doctor, and within days I saw the first of several physicians. The doctor who did the first clinical breast exam felt no lumps, acknowledged it seemed like a mastitis infection, and prescribed antibiotics. She suggested a follow up in two or three weeks, "if it does not clear up." I asked about mastitis, because usually it comes from breastfeeding, and these girls have been dry for 14 years!

And unconvinced of the proper medical diagnosis, I suggested the possibility of breast cancer. The doctor looked startled, dismissed me, and said, "Cancer does not appear overnight."

My Own Research

As a result of the day's experience, and unconvinced of the physician's conclusions, my own research began that evening on the internet ("Google doctor"). I input all my symptoms and up pops an article posted that same day from a research professor at the University of Michigan about inflammatory breast cancer.

His paper correlated with what I was currently experiencing, and explained how inflammatory breast cancer is not as rare as practitioners believe, because it is occasionally misdiagnosed as mastitis. In a display of unstoppable resilience that characterized my cancer journey, I picked up the phone, cold-called the researcher, and told him of my symptoms and dream.

"Dreams are very credible," the researcher said. "Do everything you can. Your life depends on it!"

Encouraged by this dream validation and exchange, an appointment was made with yet another doctor. Again, I made a case for inflammatory breast cancer, which was again dismissed in favor of a mastitis diagnosis. "Inflammatory breast cancer is rare. Cancer and tumors take years to develop. If you were my mother or sister, I would tell you the same thing. Just take the antibiotic," the doctor said.

This time I believe I went mad-dog, used some profanities, and told him, "No! You have to research this! It could be breast cancer!" Then I just blurted out, "Look, I have dreams that have always guided me in troubled times, ever since I was a little girl. Please, I'm trying to save my life! I was told I need to have a punch biopsy and an ultrasound because sometimes you don't see inflammatory breast cancer on a mammogram, which I had nine months ago."

I think I used more colorful language and said, "Damn it! Do your research. If I had mastitis, I would have a high temperature." Upset, I left his office because my heart-wrenching appeal got me nowhere. No better off than before

I came, with a burning, seeping anger, I thought, "Okay! I will just call every damn doctor in my medical group."

However, that proved unnecessary because in a surprising reversal of events, the doctor I blew up on earlier that day had second thoughts and called when I got home. It turned out that after my consultation, he had done some research and agreed I should have a diagnostic mammogram after all.

Although my battle for a radiology referral was won, my optimism was diminished by the threat of further delay. "The soonest they can see you is next month," the radiology receptionist informed me. I tautly pleaded for a closer appointment date. "Look, I can't just knock people off the schedule for you," was her curt reply.

By now, accustomed to challenging medical authority I countered with, "No, you don't understand. You need to do that because I might have a severe breast cancer."

The receptionist phoned the following morning with an appointment for two days later. I greeted her with flowers.

My mammogram was determined to be "unremarkable," and I was told to go home. That did it! Holding onto the seat of my chair with both hands to make my plans to go nowhere perfectly clear, I cried, "No, no! You need to do a punch biopsy and an ultrasound." Like Kat, in Chapter 2, my bold self-advocacy paid off again. The doctor relented.

Despite their tight schedule that day, the center agreed to do an ultrasound in four hours. My wait was longer. About 30 women passed through those doors before I was called, during the last office hour. The ultrasound revealed a cluster. The doctor called me back into his office to discuss the finding and told me, "You need a needle biopsy."

"I want a punch biopsy! A needle biopsy is an insufficient diagnostic tool for inflammatory breast cancer."

I said, "Are you sure this isn't inflammatory breast cancer, specifically?"

I needed the doctor to prove me wrong, and only a punch biopsy could do that.

"I have seen inflammatory breast cancer. It is rare," he replied. When I mentioned the researcher who said it is often misdiagnosed as mastitis, the doctor sitting before me pointed and said, "Do you see those degrees on that wall?"

It occurred to me that the radiologist treated what had happened today as unremarkable. He had told me to go home after a clean mammogram. When I resisted and ultimately prevailed, he ordered an ultrasound, which revealed potential abnormalities. He was concerned enough to order a biopsy. And yet, he had not the slightest curiosity about how I knew I needed to keep pushing for more accurate tests to save my life. The doctor thought it was just another busy day at the office, and now it was time to remind the patient who was the doctor, close shop, and go home.

I got the punch biopsy.

The Night Before My Biopsy I Had a Dream

I fell into a killer whale tank and was yelling for someone to please help me! The massive black-and-white beasts were slowly circling around me. At that moment, a tall, handsome man wearing a wetsuit jumped in and hugged me to him. Then one of the smaller killer whales pushed us onto the landing where we were safe.

I woke up that morning in a very positive mood, danced around the kitchen floor, and told my husband and daughter about the dream, thinking, "Yes! I'm going to live!" I told them I knew it to be true because I dove deep into whale symbolism dreams.

To me, the appearance of whales suggests something enormous is happening in the dreamer's life. And yet, here is a smaller sub-aspect of that enormity, symbolized by the little whale, which suggested I was safe no matter what. This dream was a turning point for me. Gone was my sense of dread.

A week later I was diagnosed with DCIS (ductal carcinoma in situ), multifocal and multicentric. Then it changed to grade 3 after an MRI.

The good news is it was not aggressive invasive cancer, but early stage 0 breast cancer. Though cancer is always a scary word, stage 0 in situ cancer patients, when treated, have a survival rate close to 100 percent. However, grade 3 tumors are high proliferating. Was the stage **0** the little orca? Dreams are amazing!

Had that cluster been left to fester, my cancer may have been found at a later stage, requiring more aggressive treatment. I'm grateful for those mysterious external symptoms that mimicked inflammatory breast cancer. The big red dot and deep pain kept me pushing for further screenings. Unless there is a palpable lump, which I also did not have, DCIS is often asymptomatic. An excellent prognosis and chemo-less recovery notwithstanding, my finish line was still not in sight.

Since cluster tumors have a greater likelihood of returning, three cancer doctors recommended a unilateral mastectomy. This gave me no peace of mind. If this cancer was not going to kill me, then why must I do this? Why not just do a lumpectomy and radiation like so many other breast cancer patients—some with even more advanced cancers than mine?

"It can be harder to get clean margins on multifocal tumors," the doctors said. "If cells were left behind, cancer could come back." I chose to accept their explanation and focused on finding the best surgeon to reconstruct my breast without using anything artificial.

Despite the positive aspects of the diagnosis and potential outcome, the information hit me harder than expected, possibly because my dad had just died three weeks before my diagnosis. Now, while still grieving for Dad, I had to deal with my own mortality.

I had just passed 50 years of age and started menopause. Like menopause, the diagnosis of losing my breast was another change of life, another transition. And, although I did not realize it at the time, that year would be packed full of transitions and life changes.

My goal was to feel strong during this ordeal. But bad things kept happening. Writing helped me focus on figuring out where this journey was taking me, and how to get there without losing my mind.

Dr. Larry Burk's Breast Cancer Warning Dreams Project

Once the DCIS was found, I still had to go through the big surgery of a mastectomy. But the universe had a plan. A month before his research was ending, I Googled "breast cancer dreams and women who had dreams of breast cancer before they were diagnosed." The articles found were about Kat's book and Dr. Burk's research on a dream blog.

I have always had pretty intense dreams, which have guided me during hard times. Dr. Burk talks about symbolic meaning in illness. I think you can see this in my second dream, the one with the orcas, which was really powerful. The strong orca dream really centered me and made me feel like I had a plan.

After surgery, my naturally reconstructed breast looked exactly like the other breast. Once physically recovered, healing my mental and emotional selves was my next priority. This was accomplished by participating in retreats with other cancer survivors. It helped integrate my trauma with routine aspects of life. Together, we laughed, cried, and received counseling from trained professionals. And, when it was time to move on from my cancer experience, I explored additional healing modalities.

When I look back at that time of my life, it would have been much more difficult without the help I received from positive medical people, other cancer survivors, and trained professionals. Four weeks after my breast cancer diagnosis my father had died. Then, within a year of my recovery, my mother and brother died. I had to deal with family grief while trying to stay positive and face my fears, battles, and continued healing.

My Life Had Felt Like Quicksand

To get to where I am today—healthy, confident, and writing my story for you—I got quiet within myself, journaled, and wrote down all my dreams. I came to an important conclusion.

Life is a continual journey. I transferred my focus from grief and fear to the next path along the trail of wholeness by incorporating more yoga; Eastern medicine healing philosophy; nutrition, such as drinking green tea; acupuncture therapy; meditation retreats; and writing in my daily journal. It helped me shift my focus from death and dying to breath and living. The resilience forged from my cancer crucible still guides me. Before cancer, I think I would have gotten stuck in sorrow after losing my father, brother, and mother. But after cancer, I realize life is a journey. Always! You just have to keep going.

My Learning Experiences

As far as the learning experiences I encountered, always take each day with a long, slow breath. Be grateful to be breathing. Seek out new experiences. Live life, and be with people who make you laugh. From all these life experiences I became resilient and durable. In 2013, I completed a 200-hour yoga alliance teacher training. Yoga and meditation saved me. My desire is to work with cancer survivors in the future, because (ha ha) I'm a force of nature, or so I've been told!

KAT'S INTERPRETATION

Thank goodness Diane is such a strong force of nature. Yes! Like a number of women in the study, it took effort, time, and a few tantrums for Diane to convince her physicians to perform the tests her dreams and body were telling her she needed. Diane understood her dreams quite well. If they were my dreams, I would define them as both active and symbolic diagnostic dreams validated by pathology reports. The first literal diagnostic dream used conversation with a family member. The second dream used symbolism.

The little orca was not only helpful to Diane by pushing her to safety but the first letter of the word orca is the letter which looks like the number zero; her level of cancer and the orcas circled in the tank creating another "0," known as the circle of life.

At the time, she had the dream of the little orca, she did not know her cancer would be stage 0. In the symbolic world of dreams, orcas, unlike fish, are very intelligent mammals with strong family ties. They have mammary glands or breasts like humans but are also in the water world of spirituality. Although danger existed from these circling larger mammals, the circle created the protective circle of life.

All this symbolism begs the question, who was the tall, handsome man in the wetsuit? Was he Diane's alter ego, an inner guide who came to her rescue, or someone still to be met in the future? Thank goodness Diane self-advocated, because without her inner strength we may not have had the privilege of hearing her dream story.

DR. BURK'S COMMENTARY

Diane's story is similar to that of the other Diane, in Chapter 1, my friend who insisted on an ultrasound when the mammogram was negative. Although ultrasound is not as sensitive as mammography in most cases, in women with dense breasts, it can provide valuable additional screening information. If the dream guidance is strong enough, it can give you the confidence to pursue the diagnosis more aggressively than what would be routinely done by most clinicians. MRI scans may provide even more accurate information about the extent of the tumor, so in some cases, the intuitive dream information and imaging data can be synergistic, reminding us to use the best of both worlds.

10

The Nightmare/Dream
Began on a Beautiful Fall Day...

Sunni Ingalls

*"Listening to your intuition is so important. Don't dismiss
dreams or feelings that are strong or stick with you."*

NOTE: In 2014, Sunni's story was shared in the
Huffington Post article "I Believe a Dream Saved My Life: A Tale of
Breast Cancer Detection."

I am married with two boys and live in Webster, New York. My family in the area is small but close. My job is system analyst for East Irondequoit Central School District, but after cancer treatment, I returned to work part-time. I am also a certified yoga instructor and teach one to four classes a week. On a personal note, practicing yoga changed my life and has really helped me to hone my intuition.

A Family History of Breast Cancer

We do have a family history of breast cancer, but the women in my family were diagnosed in their 50s and 60s. So only being in my early 40s gave me no concerns about my breast health, at least not yet. Additionally, my lifestyle was relatively healthy. My weight was good, I ran for exercise, and didn't eat a ton of "bad" food. But my stress levels were high!

My two teenage boys at home kept me running from one event to another while dealing with typical teenage behavior. My business had failed a few years earlier, and I really felt my current job was too demanding. Although I was not a priority in my own life, I don't think I really recognized it at the time.

Running for My Life

My breast cancer dream began on a beautiful fall day. I could feel my heart pounding and the sound of my shallow but rhythmic breathing buzzing in my ears. My entire body vibrated each time my foot struck the ground. This was

81

the day! I was in the zone! For the first time ever in my running career, I was at the front of the pack, and nothing was going to stop me! The wind was at my back, and the strength I felt was undeniable. This was the day I would set a PR! (running lingo for personal record.)

Running along, I am suddenly yanked from my thoughts by the sound of a car riding beside the race. I try to put on my blinders and concentrate on my run, but someone is calling my name. Finally, I give up and look over. I have to do a double take because it is my husband driving and waving me over like a madman!

He is pleading with me to get into the car, but I tell him he is crazy, that today is the day I am going to set a PR, and there is NO way I am leaving! We bicker for a bit and then with a promise that he will be able to return me to the same place in the race (for some reason this makes sense to me at the time), I relent and get in the car with him.

We arrive home. Upon entering, I immediately observe my reflection in the mirror. I look exhausted, and my left gland is severely swollen. I become aware of my mother's presence as she stands to the right of me with a worried look on her face.

"Mom, I will be fine."

Then, suddenly, the dream is over.

I knew instantly this was no ordinary dream and immediately called my mom, shared the dream, and explained to her something was going to happen that would "take me out of the race of life," but I was certain that "I would get right back in where I left off."

But how? Only one thing seemed obvious: whatever it was had also happened to my mother. That is why Mom was also reflected in the mirror. I was a reflection of her because my neck was swollen and my mother had thyroid issues, so I initially thought it might be that. However, my mother had also had breast cancer.

After a mammogram and subsequent ultrasound, a biopsy was taken. The doctor called me with the results the next day: invasive ductal carcinoma grade 2 breast cancer, relatively fast-growing in the left breast. My mother had been diagnosed with breast cancer years prior. Coincidence? I think not.

A Crisis of Faith

Between diagnosis and tumor staging, I had my first ever crisis of faith. Never one to doubt the existence of God or an afterlife, I was now shaken. What if this is it? What if I die and no longer exist? "Tell me I will live. Tell me I will live!" I pleaded with my husband.

General optimism that my outcome would mirror the dream never could banish all doubt. You see, anticipation of the next scan or biopsy induces being hunted in the wild, primal terror, a fight-or-flight anxiety that is only relieved by good news. Between tests and results lies Hell on Earth. However, unrelenting affirmation of what my sleeping self knew managed to keep me afloat most of the time. "I will be fine" was my refrain. "The dream said I will be fine, remember?" I clung to this like a raft, maintaining stability through cancer's eye of the storm.

My decision to trust the dream guided every step forward like a mission statement. It suggested that I would ultimately be okay, but also implied my mad-dash reality must halt to a full stop first. Accepting those terms, I took leave from my job before even having a treatment plan.

Now cocooned in quiet self-reflection, I could take stock of the life that got me here: failed business, demanding job, teenager-versus-Mom drama, racing from one responsibility to another. I was not a priority in my own life, and the consequences of this finally caught up with me. That had to change, because even if I beat this cancer, resuming my harried pace might produce more illness. Only a complete lifestyle change could restore my health.

Sensing fulfillment of the dream's promise required something new of me, retreat from the well-meaning advice of others was imperative. Now the woman who ran for other people had to slow down for herself. She must drop deep within, sit with her own needs, with her own fears, and learn the unique healing language of her own being.

Only breaking routine far from the comfort zone of my hard-pressed life could accomplish this. Not "far," as in the next state over. Not "far," as in a quiet beach on the opposite coast. South of the equator "far," to Abadiania, the remote Brazilian village where John of God is found.

The Healing Trip to John of God

John of God is an unassuming Brazilian farmer who reportedly channels spiritual entities for healing in his spare time. Thousands, including Oprah, have visited Casa de Dom de Loyola, John's healing center, nestled amid the rolling hills of central Brazil. I wanted my Casa experience to orient me toward recovery. After my treatment, if there were any disease lingering in my body, perhaps this trip might heal it, but even if it could not, I could still heal mentally and spiritually there. One way or another, I would return home whole.

Upon arrival, we said a prayer of introduction. Overcome with emotion, I felt a hand on mine. When I opened my eyes, nobody was there.

The trip was a meditative experience, drawing us deep within. There are a number of current rooms at the Casa where visitors, all dressed in white, sit in prayer and meditation to help maintain a current of energy that benefits those seeking who seek to heal. Holding space for others in the current room, we'd meditate for over three hours per stretch.

Psychic surgeries are the popular draw to John of God, as many people seek miraculous cures of their illnesses. In most cases, these are energetic in nature and not knife-to-skin procedures. My first "surgery" took place in the third current room with 30 other people. When the entities began their work, I felt movement at the base of my skull, then upward along my right side, moving to the left temple. My chest area also tingled, as did my right knee and hip. Surgery complete, I entered a 24-hour period of silence.

After surgeries and silence, attendants can engage in other integral aspects of the Casa journey, such as the pilgrimage to the Sacred Waterfall. Walking down toward the cascade felt familiar, like I had done this before. As we waited in single file along a bridge-like structure for our turns under the rushing water, a small, colorful butterfly made its way down the line, landing on almost everyone. Anxiously awaiting my turn to be selected by this exquisite creature, I was disappointed when it flew away several souls ahead of me. I felt rejected, as if the butterfly did not find me worthy.

Approaching my turn to enter this gushing tumble of water over rock, Josie, a Casa guide, led me in with a few instructions.

"Be sure you get completely wet. Run the water directly on any areas of concern. And make sure to release anything that no longer serves you."

Easier said than done, I thought. But I had noticed Josie trying to help others from her spot on the water's edge, arms moving in rhythmic motion. Maybe this was some shamanic ritual in which she assisted their release, and she would help me, too. I gasped for air as the thick, freezing water hit me. From the hollowed-out space, my body carved into the center of the fall. I heard the faint sound of my own moans. Remembering Josie's instructions, alone in this foreign land, under a crush of cold water, I released my bundle of burdens into a flood of emotion and tears. I emerged grateful for having gotten wet and hoped the droplets around my eyes might be mistaken for the fall's water.

"That was really powerful for you," said Josie. "While you were under the falls there were two blue morpho butterflies circling you. They are rare this time of year."

Boxing Up Emotional Items

During the 24-hour silent period after my second surgery, I penetrated some dark inner spaces, symbolically boxing up emotional items that no longer served me. Then after tying each package neatly with a ribbon and placing them on a raft, I set the contents ablaze and pushed the float out to sea. Mother Nature would take it from there.

In some ways, I no longer shared the priorities of the woman who boarded that plane for Brazil. I reentered my day-to-day reality committed to slowing down, forever altering how my body moves through life. For years, running was my primary exercise passion while yoga existed in the background. No mere jogger, my sneakers hit the pavement for accomplishment, races, and personal bests; yoga was just stretches I did to warm up for my true love.

These days I still run, but just for the sheer enjoyment of it. I go out now to connect, preferring trail runs in nature to concrete, asphalt, and cheers from the sidelines. Yoga, with its deep breaths and silent spaces, has emerged as my lifestyle of choice. I took yoga instructor training and now teach mindful movement to others.

Between breath and movement is life, which I now engage differently from before cancer. I emerged from illness to find my children flourishing into adult lives.

Before Cancer Versus After Cancer

I know me. Prior to having cancer, an empty nest would have riddled me with insecurity; my children taking their necessary steps toward independence would have been interpreted as a personal rejection. I can see it now. *When are you coming home to visit? What, that far from now? Well, don't bother then!* But, none of that happened. When abandonment emotions do surface, I recognize them for what they are: typical aspects of empty-nest syndrome and not the end of the world.

My cancer was a gift—mentally, physically, and spiritually. A gift I never want to have to open again, but a gift just the same. At first, I didn't tell the physicians or staff about my dream, but down the road, I shared it with one of my oncologists and my doctor at the breast clinic. Both are open-minded and encouraged me to continue to listen to my intuition and pay attention to my dreams.

Dr. Larry Burk's Dream Study

One day during my treatment, my mom sent me a link to a dream website and encouraged me to post my dream. She thought it'd be therapeutic and a great idea to get feedback on what others thought. It was the only time I had ever shared a dream on a website. I really don't normally do stuff like that. Dr. Burk contacted me from there, and that is how I became included in his study on breast cancer dreams.

Listening to your intuition is so important. Don't dismiss dreams or feelings that are strong or stick with you. That's how I describe my "prophetic/message" dreams. Take time and just sit with the thought or dream. Don't attach to it, but ask yourself some questions, like if you should act on it, follow up with a doctor, and so on, then honor yourself by following through with what you decide.

KAT'S INTERPRETATION

What an amazing healing dream story. Illness affects the whole family and shakes belief systems to their core. If this were my dream I would say it was an active diagnostic dream and, like Diane's dream, full of signs, symbols, and abstract information that made sense to the dreamer in the dream world but required deciphering in the waking world, which Sunni did beautifully.

Every dream is as individual as the dreamer who dreamt it. Sunni was in a race for her life, which was joined as a parallel adventure by her husband in the family car. A car is often considered our body in dream symbolism, so a family car might be seen as a life shared with significant others. A *mirror* in a dream can signify a need for self-reflection or a period of reflection to recognize who you are, or what you should be doing. Her reflectiveness was part of Sunni's search for self, which was begun during her journey to John of God, and is still happening today.

DR. BURK'S COMMENTARY

I have not been to visit John of God, but I have many friends who have made the pilgrimage described by Sunni. As she mentioned, he is famous for doing psychic surgery with unsterilized instruments that miraculously cause no infection or pain due to the shared hypnotic trance state of the healer and healee. However, as she points out, much of healing occurs on an internal level in the energetic "current" of the Casa.

Her description of nurturing everyone else while failing to adequately nurture herself is a common theme among breast cancer patients, as mentioned previously with Amparo. It is a classic earth element imbalance, impacting the breast through the stomach meridian. In order to address this issue, which is usually invisible to the conscious mind, Sunni had to be taken out of the race in her dream.

Thankfully, she got the message loud and clear and made the self-nurturing decisions necessary to heal. It often does take radical steps to create a *Radical Remission*, the title of the best-selling book by oncology psychotherapist Kelly Turner, which I recommend to all my cancer patients. It documents the stories of stage 4 cancer patients who were sent to hospice but then wound up alive and well many years later. She identified nine different common themes of lifestyle changes used by these miraculous spontaneous remitters, including one with a malignant brain tumor who spent many months with John of God before returning home completely healed.

11

My Dream Doctor is Real

Denise

*"When I wake up I realize the dream is telling me I need a
mastectomy because my body is full of foreign cells."*

My name is Denise. I am 67 years of age and semi-retired from a 24-year career in health care. In 2001, for our 20th anniversary, my husband and I took a vacation to Canada. From the beginning, it did not seem right or comfortable.

I Have a Dream

A month or so after returning from our trip, I had a disturbing dream.

> In the dream, I am speaking with an old friend, Adam, who has had several episodes of a rare and unusual cancer. I have just been diagnosed with an early form of cancer and am a bit freaked out. So I ask him what kind of advice he can give me to deal with this. In the background, I hear a woman physician (who I do not recognize from waking life) saying to me, "Don't worry, Denise, we have lots of ways of dealing with this."

A few months later, I have my annual mammogram. The radiologist tells me that they see something "suspicious" and suggests a biopsy. The radiologist is the same person who always looks at my mammogram films. He shows me the odd-looking calcifications in the left breast. Calcifications are routinely seen in my right breast, but this time there are some in the left. These calcifications appear different, so the radiologist recommends a biopsy.

"What is the worst-case scenario?" I ask.

To which he says, "DCIS, which is ductal carcinoma in situ."

My Dream Doctor

I start interviewing surgeons, and the second one is a woman who really clicks with me. Driving home in the car I tell my husband, "I am going with this doctor. She feels right." A few minutes later, I turn to my husband and say, "Oh my. She was the physician in my dream!"

Dodging a Bullet

That night I have a second dream.

> In the dream, I am the passenger in a car with a friend, driving out into the countryside for some kind of gathering. All of a sudden, I see a car racing down the dirt road, and the driver is shooting at people. Some of the people are running, some are getting shot, some are diving under their cars. I watch the car stop about 50 feet in front of us and feel the need to hide from him. I scrunch down underneath the dashboard, and he drives by without stopping or shooting.

Upon awakening I say to my husband, "I've dodged a bullet." My dream told me I dodged a health bullet that was a real killer.

It was a very hectic time that summer, as my in-laws were planning a big 50th-anniversary celebration in the Midwest and we were trying to get organized to attend. I had one biopsy with the surgeon, and when she could not get clean margins, she did a second biopsy. She still could not get clean margins and said to me, "I'm happy to do a third biopsy, but I think it is a waste of time. A mastectomy would be our best course of action."

Foreigners Help Me in a Dream

At that point, I had a third dream.

> I am visiting relatives in another state for a cousin's wedding and am in the townhouse of that cousin. But nowhere in the townhouse is anyone I recognize. It is all foreign people from South America, from Europe, from the Middle East, and from Asia, from the attic to the basement. They are not destructive, tearing down walls or even dangerous. They are just everywhere.

I wake up and tell my husband, "I need to have a mastectomy." It is clear to me that the dream is saying a mastectomy is the only answer because my body is full of foreign cells.

Throughout this entire journey, I felt many emotions: anger, sadness, disappointment, resentment, frustration, grief, and aggravation. The one emotion missing was fear.

I have been a fearful person most of my life. Most people would not know that about me as it is hidden well. The most amazing gift about these dreams was they told me from the first day I had nothing to fear. They reassured me and gave me direction. I was quite happy about this and moved through the experience with no real worries about the outcome.

My late sister even remarked to me, "I was getting freaked out because you were not freaked out." To which I said, "Karen, I have been keeping a dream journal since 1984, and my dreams have never lied to me."

Every healthcare practitioner I met was told about my dreams, and all were quite supportive. No one dismissed them or suggested they were irrelevant. In fact, every year during my follow-up visit my surgeon routinely asks, "Have you had any more dreams about me?"

Dr. Larry Burk's Dream Study Group

I heard about Dr. Larry Burk's study group either online, on the IASD's website, or perhaps on Facebook. Jeremy Taylor has been my teacher, mentor, and inspiration since the first workshop I took with him in 1995. He is one of the original four founders of the International Association for the Study of Dreams (IASD). I took every workshop I could with him and found his work to be fabulously inspiring, interesting, and extremely valuable. I worked with my dreams a little bit with a therapist I had seen, and always had a deep interest in dreams.

His workshops helped me understand the incredible value to be found in listening to our dreams and making space to hear what they might be telling us. I am now a certified dreamwork facilitator and have led workshops and many dream groups in the area where I live.

KAT'S INTERPRETATION

Denise is a master at her own dream language explanations and was able to understand the messages immediately upon waking. If her first dream had been mine, I would have classified it as a literal diagnostic dream for a number of reasons. The doctor in the dream used Literal words to reassure Denise that she had options, and the doctor in the dream was her future doctor, whom she had not yet met. Therefore, the dream was precognitive and did come true.

If her second dream were mine, I would define it as a Symbolic Informative Dream because she "dodged a *bullet*" (deadly cancer) from a *speeding car*, which may have been her speeding life at that time. She did not panic like the other people in her dream, but rather chose to "hunker down under the *dashboard*," where there are computers, wires to the radio, and the communication part or healing right brain of the car to save herself in the dream, and also in her waking future. If her third dream were mine, I would describe it as a symbolic diagnostic dream because a *house* is a body. Her body was invaded by "foreign bodies," top to bottom.

DR. BURK'S COMMENTARY

Meeting future healthcare practitioners in dreams seems to a common precognitive theme for several of the breast cancer dreamers, including my friend Diane, Suzanne, and now Denise. Dreams that are that vividly real do instill a sense of confidence that the rest of the dream guidance for healing will also be right. It is of particular importance when needing to trust the intuitive information in making challenging decisions, such as whether to have a mastectomy or not. Of course, having decades of experience dream journaling certainly does provide a sound basis for knowing how to use dreams when you need them. Hopefully, this book will inspire its readers to follow suit.

12

Transcending Breast Cancer: Reconstructing One's Self

Carolyn K. Kinney, PhD, RN

"There is an invisible world and a spiritual presence available to us all the time. We just need to be open to this presence."

This chapter is part of a larger professional article written by the author about her in-depth personal journey through and beyond breast cancer. The article can be read in its entirety at *Issues in Mental Health Nursing*. 17:201-216, 1996.

M y story begins with an event that occurred one mid-August afternoon. Two evenings prior, I had returned from the memorial service held for my younger brother, who had died unexpectedly. I was desperately in need of physical, emotional, and spiritual renewal and decided to lie down for a short nap.

The Dream Message

After about 45 minutes of surprisingly deep, and restful sleep...

> I was floating in that foggy in-between place, starting to wake up but still mostly asleep. A message came to me so loudly and clearly that it instantly jolted me out of the fog. So vivid, it was as if simultaneously I heard, felt, and perhaps even saw the command: go make your appointment for your mammogram right now. Do not delay.

A little shaken but trying to keep grounded, I found myself on the phone asking the receptionist at the mammography center for the next available appointment. I explained that my yearly gynecological examination was scheduled for the following Tuesday, and it would be helpful to have the mammography results at that time.

She exclaimed, "You've got to be kidding. I'm sure we won't have anything that soon." Then, she put me on hold to take another call, and in about half a minute she returned to say, "Well, this is your lucky day. That was a cancellation. You can come in at 2 p.m. on Monday."

As I hung up the phone, I had both a feeling of urgency about the task at hand and some apprehension about the outcome, but the more prevailing feeling that settled in was one of calmness. I had a sense of comfort that I was doing what needed to be done and things would work out alright.

Thus Began My Journey Through and Beyond Breast Cancer

The dream reconnected me with an experience I had as I returned from the memorial service for Nick and a compassionate stranger who helped me through my grief. All I wanted was to get home and catch a quick nap while on the airplane. I sat down in the first available aisle seat, and even before the plane had taken off I had dropped into a deep sleep. Thirty minutes later I was awakened by the pilot's voice saying our landing would be delayed due to a thunderstorm hovering over the airport in Austin. "It's just decided to hang around for a while," the pilot explained with a chuckle.

A man sitting next to me was looking out the window and remarked about how thrilling it was to see a thunderstorm from this vantage point. He alerted some boys sitting behind him to "catch the view" out the window and told them it was a rare sight they might really enjoy. I remember thinking, *How refreshing to hear someone so thrilled by an act of nature.* My mind briefly toyed with the idea that this man's enthusiasm was so much like Nick's. I looked at him more closely and realized he even looked like Nick. His mustache, his build, his gestures, his laugh, and his friendly manner all reminded me of Nick. I dismissed these thoughts, however, saying quietly, "It is just because you miss him so much."

The pilot again announced that the thunderstorm was still "hanging around" and we would circle Austin for about 30 more minutes, but if unable to land by then we would need to return to Dallas. I exclaimed something like, "Oh for crying out loud. This is ridiculous."

The man said, "You know, I've flown a lot through the years, and it's amazing this has never happened to me. Hopefully, it isn't a real problem for you. Are you going to a funeral or something like that?"

I shook my head and said, "No, no, I'm not going to a funeral." I hesitated and thought, "Why should I explain to him what is going on in my life. He is only a stranger." Then I realized he was reaching out to me in a kind rather than nosy manner. I reconsidered and said, "I'm coming back from one."

"I thought so. You look so sad."

Surprised by his perceptiveness, I said, "Really?"

"Yes, I could tell something was really troubling you. Tell me about it. I'm serious. I don't have anything else to do right now. We're stuck here on the plane, and I'm concerned and interested."

I felt I could trust him and proceeded to describe Nick, share some of his life, and express how difficult it had been for my whole family, including my father and older brother. My mother had already passed from breast cancer.

He looked at me with such sincere knowing in his gentle brown eyes. "Tell me about your fondest memories. I'll understand. I've lost loved ones, too."

I shared happy memories, some funny incidents, and a few typical Nick stories. We laughed and even cried together on that plane in the thunderstorm.

After 30 minutes, I was feeling considerably better and told him how much I appreciated his interest and concern. Hesitatingly, I reached out to touch him, and he extended his hand to me. Rather than a handshake, our hands came together in an overlapping grip that felt so secure and familiar.

We made eye contact, and he said, "Thank you for telling me about Nick. I know you two were very close. I've learned a lot from our conversation, and it has helped me, too."

At that instant, the pilot announced the storm had moved on, and we were cleared for landing.

Despite the many ways this compassionate stranger reminded me of Nick, my rational mind dismissed the experience as merely a very nice man who reached out to me in a time of need. However, two days later, after the phone call scheduling my mammogram, I awoke in the middle of the night with a different interpretation.

I heard myself asking, "Could the stranger on the plane be Nick?" Tears streamed down my face as my inner voice answered the question with a resounding "Yes." As if to affirm this to be true, I remembered immediately upon hearing of Nick's death I had expressed the wish, "If only I could see him and touch him one more time."

My encounter with the compassionate stranger gave me that opportunity to see and touch him one more time. I am comforted by the belief that Nick's spirit stayed on this earthly plane long enough to console me and perhaps be consoled by me. The experience has been the key to my sense of transcendence; it has given me peace and comfort and has opened the door to how I might place my life within a bigger picture.

The Foreshadowed Test

A few days later, I went to my mammography appointment with mixed emotions, both saddened and energized by the recent events and dreams. I was full of wonder and in awe of what life can bring. Given the excitement and mystery surrounding the making of the appointment, I prepared myself for the possibility that it might turn out to be something other than a routine mammogram.

It was not routine. Several retakes of the mammogram were required. The magnification needed to be increased a second and then a third time. Microcalcifications were present in my left breast, and a biopsy was scheduled for that Friday.

Gathering Information

To prepare for my biopsy, I started gathering information and rallying support from a variety of sources. I talked with family and friends and alerted them to what was happening and asked for their thoughts and prayers. I spent time praying, meditating, and reflecting on my encounter with the compassionate stranger. This experience was life-changing. It provided me with a view beyond the visible world[52] and reconfirmed for me that there is an invisible world and a spiritual presence available to us all the time. We just need to be open to this presence. Further, I realized I had many sources of spiritual support and comfort into which I could tap. I also reaffirmed the continual presence in my life of people who were significant sources of support in my past but were no longer living.

One such reaffirmation occurred just a few days before Nick's death, when I happened upon a picture of my mother stored away in a drawer. Immediately upon making my discovery, I strategically placed it in clear view on a marble-topped antique table in my dining room. Mother's presence was palpable and gave me much comfort during those initial days following Nick's death and later during my cancer treatment.

A second example of unexpected and unplanned reconnection with family from my past occurred at a Christmas bazaar. While not looking for anything in particular, I stopped cold and suspended in motion as a pair of grandmother and grandfather ceramic dolls looking so much like my deceased grandparents caught my attention. I placed my treasured grandparent dolls by the fireplace in my living room. Intuitively, I was surrounding myself with supportive images and icons in preparation for the dark days to come.

There were many difficult times during these days of waiting, but the worst one was waiting for the biopsy results. The longer I waited, the more anxious I became and lost touch with my sense of calmness.

The call finally came, and my surgeon reported that I had two types of cancer, lobular and intraductal. Both were in situ, and this fact was certainly in my favor. However, hearing that I had cancer put me in a state of shock.

Due to the early nature of the disease process, the recommended treatment approaches ranged from "do nothing further" to bilateral mastectomies with potential follow-up chemotherapy or radiation and various combinations of possible options in between. Before I hung up the phone with my surgeon, I heard myself say, "I think the thing to do is go ahead with the bilateral mastectomies."

This precipitous pronouncement surprised me because my mother had been diagnosed with breast cancer in 1960, and at that time the only option available to her was a radical mastectomy. I had seen her go through that extensive and body-altering surgery and was perplexed and distraught when she died a little more than two years later.

Even before my diagnosis, my mother's experience had led me to think rather often about what I might do if I had breast cancer. I considered the various treatment alternatives developed in recent years and, in the abstract, had concluded a mastectomy would not be my choice. Yet, when faced with the real decision, my inner voice was saying not just one but two.

The final decision was consistent with my initial response. I came to see that losing my breast or breasts was far less threatening than losing my life.

While meditating one morning a day or two before surgery, I heard my inner voice say, "When I return from surgery, it will be the same me. I'll just have some of my parts rearranged." I repeated this mantra to my family as I was wheeled into the operating room.

Two days later, the pathology report indicated no further cancer cells were found and the oncologist said no follow-up medical treatment was required. This was excellent news.

I now realize that by the time I went to surgery I was well along my path to transcendence. My view of my self had changed. I had known that the physical self is essential and must be listened to, attended to, and cared for. However, as I had progressed in my spiritual exploration and growth, I came to embrace more fully that there is so much more to me than my physical body. The physical self may be the visible self; however, it is the invisible self that is really what is real.

Moving on with an Inner Voice

Listening to my inner voice has provided me with a sense of connection with an inner and outer source of wisdom and caring. Messages have come in various forms, sometimes as a voice speaking to me as I am aroused from sleep, such as the mammogram appointment command. At other times, I have sought guidance through specific questions or requests posed during my prayers and meditations. Still other times, I have experienced a sense of intuitive knowing that has led me to do something that just feels right, even though I may not fully know why. Throughout this story, there are many examples of how I benefited from heeding the guidance of my inner voice.

Breast cancer has been an incredible journey; one of darkness and light, fear, and love, sadness, and joy. It has been a lonely voyage, at times, but I know that I have not done it alone. I have had the love, help, and support of people very dear to me, both living and deceased. And, the inner voice that took me to the phone that August afternoon has endured.

Dr. Larry Burk's Dream Study

I became aware of Dr. Larry Burk's Breast Cancer Dreams Project through my former School of Nursing dean, who knew a dream had alerted me to the possibility of breast cancer. She heard about the project from Larry Dossey, contacted me and, in turn, I contacted Dr. Burk and joined his project.

KAT'S INTERPRETATION

If this were my dream, like Carolyn, I would have embraced and heeded that inner voice in the diagnostic dream. Although Carolyn did not describe symbolism in her dream, it may have been an extension of her inner voice that told her to make a mammography appointment "without delay." Like Paulette's and my dreams, Carolyn's guided dream was Audio (the use of specific words) rather than Symbolic (the use of signs and symbols that require interpretation). No mistake could be made in the dream's interpretation. This is a perfect example of how a dream can be instrumental in the early detection of cancer. The earlier the cancer diagnosis, the better the prognosis. Her inner voice even answered questions for her concerning dreams. We are made up of much more than id, ego, and super-ego. We have many invisible inner selves which, when working together with our visible "outer self," are quite powerful.

DR. BURK'S COMMENTARY

Dr. Kinney was ahead of her time in publishing her report in the nursing literature, and I am grateful to Dr. Larry Dossey for his part in facilitating our connection while I was recruiting subjects for the study. She actually brought another dreaming friend of hers along to participate as well.

Carolyn's story reminds us that sometimes the only dream recall is a powerful voice upon awakening, but it can still have as profound an effect as detailed visual experience. Several others of the dreamers in this book report a similar experience, including the woman who found her recurrent breast cancer, as told in Chapter 3.

13

She Who Dreams the
Dance of the Dead

Wanda Burch

*"It is up to the individual to turn illness into a spiritual exercise
and to bring dreams and other alternative healing methods of choice
into the healing process."*

I am an historian and writer, and in 2018, a breast cancer survivor for over 27 years. In 2003, New World Library published the story of my experience of healing and dreams, *She Who Dreams: A Journey into Healing through Dreamwork*. In the book, I describe how working with dreams and dream imagery saved my life—not a process of one dream, but a process that involved keeping a journal, working with individual dream imagery, and understanding the ongoing process of diagnosis, action, healing, and the information and imagery in each dream.

Illness, particularly cancer, on the surface does not appear to be a spiritual exercise. It has the ability to paralyze, to cause the suspension of good judgment, and to create an environment where options seem to no longer exist. When the body is dealt a severe physical blow, doctors often take advantage of the situation, providing healing options that define healing within the most narrow of definitions. It is up to the individual to turn illness into a spiritual exercise and to bring dreams and other alternative healing methods of choice into the healing process.

Healing Choices in a Haunting Recurrent Dream

I was given the opportunity of healing options over 25 years ago, when diagnosed with breast cancer. My dreams prepared me, 20 years in advance, for the challenge of a life-threatening illness. They presented, over time, a haunting recurring dream with slight changes in details to reflect my changing age.

In each of these dreams, I danced down a hallway peopled with the dead to my own death, which lay just beyond a small wooden door. In the last of the dance hall dreams, I wore a wedding gown, a bride dancing to her appointment with death, and was presented a newspaper detailing my age: 43 years old.

It was the year of my eventual diagnosis and treatment for breast cancer. The dance hall dreams haunted me until I received a dream in the last month of my chemotherapy treatments, a dream that renewed and extended my life and my sense of purpose.

Dream visitors warned me of impending illness and finally pushed me to go to doctors before I developed physical symptoms. Specific dreams guided me in my choice of treatment and enabled me to support the medical treatments I chose and allowed me to develop a healing and creative relationship with my physicians.

In the wake of surgery, my dreams offered compelling imagery for self-healing and recovery. My adventures in dreaming took me to places of healing and transformation in a deeper reality and introduced me to spiritual guides and helpers who opened a path beyond fear and pain into transformation (see Chapter 37). My dreams gave me back my life. In dreaming, I found I was able, quite literally, to renegotiate my soul's contract. Dreams also opened me to a deeper life and gave me gifts to bring to others in everyday life.

I was born in Cullman, Alabama, and grew up in Memphis, Tennessee. My grandmother was a healer in the Alabama mountains, and dream sharing was a constant in my life. Keeping a daily journal was not a part of my life until a friend, Robert Moss, encouraged me to do so. The journal saved my life.

When I realized I was dreaming the diagnosis of breast cancer, Robert was in the process of developing a set of "questions," which he called the Lightning Dream Technique. In helping me work with and understand my night dreams, I worked through the process of diagnosis, surgery, chemotherapy, and healing, as Robert refined his technique, assisting me in learning how to mine the dreams for active work with the imagery for healing.

As I shared the story of my dreams in She Who Dreams, and how they figured in the diagnosis of my illness and the story of my journey through surgery, chemotherapy, and depression back to healing and health, I also shared the story of my family, of my grandmother, of my father's death, of a journey to Africa, and of my dreams in the year before my diagnosis and surgery. They were all part of the evolving story of my dreaming, inseparable from the story of my life.

Dreams of my father and grandmother provided me with the guidance and support only those who have passed to the other side can offer. My dad sometimes interfered with my journey. His fears and concern for me, as his child, came through in my dreaming; perhaps also his hesitancy in wondering if I had the strength to fight such a battle. His presence in my first big warning dream, in which he appeared with a doctor demanding that I seek help, foreshadowed his appearance in subsequent dreams, in which he performed the role of guardian and guide.

My grandmother played roles as guide and teacher. She defined spirit and soul for me. She brought me healing plants and provided memory so that I could reach back into my Southern past and pull forward the best of my heritage. That heritage, my roots, descended through a line of strong Scots/Irish-American women in the Alabama hills, which began in memory with my great-grandmother and gathered momentum in my important childhood dreaming.

Warning Dreams

My dreams predicting a health problem had become murky and disturbing long before I walked into a doctor's office. My understanding of those dreams was not yet in sync, until the big dream in which my father and a doctor shouted at me that I had breast cancer and was in serious trouble. I needed to find a doctor I could trust because "no one would believe me," my father warned. That dream occurred in West Africa, where I was volunteering for an archaeology Earthwatch Team in Asantemanso, in one of the most sacred places for the Asante people.

I felt compelled to go on the African journey, almost driven, as if I would find something important in the life of a people and in the culture of a community far removed from me in space and time. Dreams of packing for a journey filled my nights. However, the image of "journeying" took on a deeper dream significance. Often, there were images of packing for two trips: a mental journey and a physical journey.

Acting on dreams that frightened me but that I did not yet understand, I made an appointment with my gynecologist, despite her intense arguments that my dreaming was about drinking too much caffeine; however, my plans for my winter journey to West Africa were already solidified, and the gynecology appointment was delayed. I had tickets, shots, reading material, and was already packing and repacking, just as in my dreams, attempting to organize everything I needed into a single backpack, a requirement for this journey.

I was also preoccupied with thoughts about the lump I had already discovered in my breast, and with the pain, although I was told it was nothing and that pain was never associated with a malignancy.

I initially believed all the packing dreams were about the physical journey to Africa. The most evocative journey dreams dealt directly with images of my trip to Africa and with images of my healing journey.

Two Journeys Dream

I am packing. Someone is talking to me, telling me I am to go on two journeys, both of them important. One journey requires more preparation than the other. I find myself in the back of a large jeep, attempting to gather things together, packing and repacking. I have prepared for the trip to Africa, but I am confused. I have to repack because I have forgotten things that I need: my visa, my passport, and other documents, plus, much to my disappointment, someone is beside me, telling me I have packed for the wrong journey. Finally, everything is together for the trip to Africa. I speak to the person who is standing beside me and tell him excitedly I am ready to go to Ghana. The person is gentle. He tells me softly that, of the two journeys, the second journey is more important and involves fewer things to pack. However, he says that I should go on the journey to Ghana first, because it will prepare me for the larger journey.

The dream continued into Africa, the images of illness taking priority.

I leave the village and move to the top of a hill, walking under trees, my feet crunching something that appears to be some kind of nuts, almost peanut in shape. I have a guide with me. He tells me to open one of the nuts. I try, but there are several layers of shell. Finally, a fruit emerges but with it a worm, which is eating away at the core of the fruit. My guide tells me there is a problem with the fruit from "my" tree and that I must take care of the problem, that I must destroy the worm in the fruit before it destroys the tree. The guide tells me I must look around the tree for images that I need. He says that I am on my final stop before I begin my journey and that I must gather what I need.

In this dream, there was a direct warning of illness, a worm in the fruit (my breast) that could, without intervention, destroy the tree (my life). Intuitively I also "knew" I had breast cancer, but the medical community responded slowly, hesitantly, convinced that I was imagining a problem. I wanted to believe the dreams indicated some other problem in my life, but I knew they originated within the deepest part of my soul, someplace within myself—the doctor within—that had a profound knowledge of my physical and mental makeup.

102

Gathering "what I needed"—the tools, the images to be used in my recovery—would become another recurring theme in my dreams. These tools would be necessary in the face of such a terrifying disease.

When I returned home to upstate New York, the dream of my father and the dream of the worm in the fruit sent me to doctors' offices, where I battled for tests that would prove my dreaming and intuition accurate. A mammogram was negative; an ultrasound, at first cautiously interpreted, defined a possible problem. An astute doctor, willing to acknowledge my intuitive source, allowed me to use a dream to show him the exact location of the malignancy for a biopsy (see Chapter 1). The dream presented me with an image I could use in meditation, between that day and the first visit with my surgeon.

In finding ways to tell my story, I became a peer advocate reviewer with the Department of Defense breast cancer grant proposal program and have had articles published on dream imagery in self-help magazines, online blogs, and other similar publications. I co-present arts retreats in the Adirondack Mountains of New York State—one at Great Camp Sagamore, for women surviving chronic illness, and one at Wiawaka in Lake George, for women veterans. These are under the auspices of Creative Healing Connections, Inc.

Most recently, I have partnered with John Kenosian, singer/songwriter. We offer programs on healing through dreams and music that allow participants the opportunity to explore the imagery in their dreams and the healing potential of music. Both John and I are featured in a 2016 CD produced for the 77th NY Regimental Balladeers, "Come, Dearest, the Daylight is Gone," with an accompanying booklet authored by myself, *Dreaming of Home in the American Civil War*. The booklet includes excerpts from my newest book on the healing potential of the soldier dreaming of home: *The Home Voices Speak Louder than the Drum: Dreams and the Imagination in Civil War Letters and Memoirs* (McFarland Publishing, Inc., 2017).

Dr. Larry Burk's Dream Study

Dr. Burk contacted me sometime in 2013 or earlier, saying he was preparing a paper and had "quoted liberally from your writings and book *She Who Dreams*, so I hope I've done justice to your work." We were both participants on the DreamsCloud.com website. He shared his paper and asked for edits. Then Kelly Walden and Martha Mert contacted me with this announcement:

Larry Burk, MD, CEHP and Healing Imager, Inc., in collaboration with DreamsCloud, are seeking volunteers who have been diagnosed with breast cancer after experiencing warning dreams, to participate in a study and share their dreams. The study will help to shed light on what aspects of such dreams may be useful to healthcare professionals for the detection of breast cancer in the future... The study will be collecting data through November 22, 2013.

Larry used my story and the stories of other women to inspire other people to share their dream experiences. In 2015, Larry published a blog for Breast Cancer Awareness Month, which featured my story and that of Kathleen (Kat) O'Keefe-Kanavos from his Breast Cancer Dreams Project paper and announced that he and Kat were collaborating on a book on dreams of warning for all types of cancer.

KAT'S INTERPRETATION

Wanda understood her dream language, which gave her the information and tools to get the treatment she desperately needed to live, and heal. If these were my dreams, I would define them as recurrent precognitive guided and diagnostic dreams showing a future event that are both literal and symbolic. They are symbolic with the Dance Hall of the Dead and the hallway in her mind with the last door of life on the end. Hallways are often areas of transition with doors as choices. "Do you want what is behind door number 1, 2, or 3 all the way at the end of this transition?"

The fruit with worms from her tree of life is also strongly symbolic, while the dated newspaper is literal within symbolism, and the conversations with her guides and deceased family are literal. Her waking daily preparations for a big journey to Africa, the seed of mankind and land of wild wonder, is again played out in a guided symbolic dream, in which the seed or peanut from her tree of life is infected with worms that are destroying the tree. This reflected her inner packing in preparation for the findings within her body and mind. These dreams were life imitating a dream imitating life. Which was the dream? Which was life?

DR. BURK'S COMMENTARY

Wanda's amazing story brings me full circle, as finding her book was what gave me the final incentive to do the project. As a professional historian, she is able to recount her own personal history in a most compelling style. It was Wanda who first brought to my attention the phenomenon of deceased relatives bringing the diagnostic information in dream form. I mentioned previously that Paulette and one other woman in the study had dreams warning them of their cancer five and nine years prior to diagnosis, but the dance hall dream was two decades prior to Wanda's breast cancer. If you read her book, you will understand that it is like her whole life has been one long dream journey, with the vital guidance and companionship of her dream teacher, Robert Moss.

14

Three Crabs, Three Pearls, and a Physician-Within

Kathleen (Kat) O'Keefe-Kanavos

Jesus said to them, "Surely you will quote this proverb to me,
'Physician, heal thyself! Do here in your hometown what
we have heard that you do in Capernaum.'"
— **LUKE 4:23**, *The Bible*

On April Fools Day, I desperately dig through my bedside dresser drawer for a pencil and paper while repeating the title for a lucid nightmare I pray is not precognitive. I've named it "Three Crabs, Three Pearls, and a Physician-within."

I enter my dream through a door into a comfortable, brightly decorated hospital waiting room and greet all the people. Some people I have met in previous dreams during my battle with breast cancer.

A happy, tall, dark-haired young woman wearing a long, colorful skirt sits on an ottoman. I don't know her name but have seen her in other dreams. She holds an adorable, diapered baby on her lap.

A door opens to the right of me, and a white-coated female physician with shoulder-length brown hair and a stethoscope draped around her neck enters the waiting room, walks up to me, holds out her hand in greeting and says, "Hi. I'm Dr. Jules (or Jewels). I'm your Physician-within."

Billy is there, too, from previous dreams. (The other teenagers in my dreams defined him to me as retarded and said due to his condition he is always honest in his questions and answers. They are very protective of him.) Billy towers over everyone and walks on the balls of his feet.

Billy asks, "Why am I here?"

Dr. Jules looks around the room and answers, "We're all here."

As if on cue, three crabs appear, scurry across the floor, and head for the basement door on the left.

"Catch them!" I hear someone yell as they pass me.

So, I give chase and keep them in sight, as they scamper down three flights of stairs toward the dark basement tunnels. If they separate and take off in different directions, it will be impossible to find them. They will grow and multiply in the dark halls. My dream has turned into a nightmare!

Frustrated, frightened, and at a loss as to what to do as they gain speed and reach the bottom step, I yell, "Stop!" I'm shocked when they obey. I quickly scoop them into a deep, clear, round plastic container filled with clear water, which materialized in my hand. As I gaze down at the submerged, contained crabs, they pull in their legs and claws and turn into three beautiful white pearls.

A lid appears in my left hand, and I put it on the on the container, and wonder as I begin to awaken, "Why are there *three* crabs? Why *three* pearls?"

I awaken shivering from fear in sweat-drenched night clothes and sopping wet hair. What the hell are three crabs doing in my dream? I have had only one stage 2 DCIS breast cancer in my right breast with one lymph node affected. Two crabs at the most! All the lymph nodes were removed. So, what am I missing? Could this dream be wrong when all the other dreams were right? If this dream is not wrong, it will be a real nightmare in my "waking world" as well.

KAT'S INTERPRETATION

This precognitive dream/nightmare deals with medical information and uses the universal symbol for cancer, *crabs*, which transform into *pearls*, beauty, and perfection through irritation. In my lucid sleep, I enter my inner realms, and I'm greeted by all the aspects of myself, including my *Physician-within*. But, I'm very concerned that there are three crabs, or cancers, and wonder about the accuracy of the information. I had a tumor in my right breast and one lymph node (two crabs?), but they were removed.

Although I don't know it at the time, this is a precognitive dream with valuable health information for the future. *A hospital room* indicates a growing state of healing consciousness. In lucid sleep, I enter my inner realm and greet all the aspects of myself, including *Dr. Jules* (doctor within, heal thyself) and *Billy*, the retarded boy from previous dreams (and most basic thoughts), and join a *young woman* (female aspect of consciousness) who holds a baby, something new like life, on her lap. *A lap* represents the first and second chakras, tribe, "gut feelings." The room is surrounded by positive feelings of the female aspects of self, which is important because it is hard to see yourself as positive and female when you lack hair and feel like shit. *The waiting room* is a play on words and reinforces "temporary."

Three symbolizes great strength and spiritual and God forces flowing through the endocrine system. The *crab* is the universal sign for cancer; the third sign of the zodiac. *Claws* are the power to hold and wound, an aspect of cancer. *Clear water* is purification and symbolizes the water of life.

A *container* does not allow something to move or spread. A top is a complete containment. *Underground passageways* are the body's basement, the subconscious mind, and the foundation of one's being, since all houses are built from the foundation up. As a duality, the passageways can also be milk ducts in breasts, where cancer often spreads. *Running* is usually away from a problem, but in my case, I run toward a problem in order to contain it.

This dream again reinforces a message by which I live: to effectively battle illness we must get in touch with our "inner selves" and work together toward the goal of survival. It shows I have the power to order cancer to stop, and it will obey.

Once the cancer is completely submerged in the clear water, it pulls in legs and claws rendering it sedate or in remission and no longer spreading. It becomes three pearls. *Pearls* represent perfection through irritation from a grain of sand-calcification. (I've certainly been irritated by this illness.) As I stare down into the container, the number three confuses me. Three crabs? Three cancers? Three pearls?

Five years later, almost to the day, the dream came true when my spirit guide monks returned and told me my cancer was back during a mammography reading, and again in a dream full of doctors dressed in clown suits. I did not want to believe the guides or dreams. I begged them to be wrong in my dreams, but realized I had to pull out my feather and use it again on my doctors because they were refusing to give me the MRI I knew I needed to find the second cancer. They still believed all mammograms worked, even though they did not find my first breast cancer.

The second breast cancer was 9 x 11 cm large. The third crab was found when changed doctors and went to New York for a double mastectomy. The third crab was found just in time; it was the end of stage 0 lobular breast cancer.

So, the Three Crabs Dream was a literal and symbolic diagnostic and precognitive dream that came true years later and was validated by multiple pathology reports. After my double mastectomy, my New York oncological surgeon said, "Kat, your dreams are going to be the talk of the New York medical society cocktail parties." I certainly hope so.

But those dreams are all about breast cancer recurrence. Perhaps that will be Dr. Larry Burk's Breast Cancer Dreams Project topic for the next book, because recurrence happens but is not a death sentence, especially when we listen to our dreams.[53]

DR. BURK'S COMMENTARY

Kat's precognitive dreams of the three crabs do raise some interesting research questions about whether dreams can accurately predict recurrence, or at the least the probability of it. One woman mentioned in Chapter 3 had her recurrence signaled upon awakening by a dream voice, even though she did not have a dream prior to her initial diagnosis. Her story may inspire other women with a history of breast cancer who read the book and are worried about recurrence to start paying attention to their dreams, even if though they have no experience with keeping a dream diary.

One theoretical concern regarding the power of the mind-body connection is whether a precognitive dream can become a self-fulfilling prophecy through creating fear and a negative impact on the immune surveillance system. Ideally, we would like all dreams to be empowering, and it is encouraging to note that the women dreamers in the study were often able to continue using their dreams for healing as is described in Part Six.

The description of the crabs turning into pearls also brings to mind the woman mentioned in Chapter 3 who proved to have a benign tumor after months of energy healing. When her dream guide said she had breast cancer, he showed her a pearl. I wonder whether that meant that the outcome would eventually be favorable in a fashion similar to Kat's healing journey, although we don't have biopsy proof of the original diagnosis. Hopefully, more research will give us insight into the diagnostic and prognostic meaning of these dream images.

15

Divorce Dream and Breast Cancer

Mary

Dr. Burk: Mary's story is included here to represent the many other women we have heard from since the original Breast Cancer Dreams Project study was published who have told us new stories about breast cancer dreams. These women provide the inspiration for future research in this area. Although there was no pathological proof, Mary's story is similar to the woman from Chapter 3 whose tumor turned out to be benign after energy healing.

KAT: This dreamer deserves a big hug for being so giving of herself by agreeing to share her awesome dreams, and that of a client, titled Mary's Client in Chapter 50, to help other people learn to understand and use their dreams for health and healing. Although we received written permission from her to use the stories, after a discussion with her children, she requested to remain anonymous, so we are respecting her wish. For the purpose of this story, we changed her name to Mary and referred to the client as Mary's Client.

I met Mary on the social media site LinkedIn, after posting about how Dr. Larry Burk and I were actively collecting stories of dreams that diagnosed illness and came true. Aside from her clinical work, Mary is an intuitive who uses regression therapy to explore dream phenomena. Mary contacted me and said she would be willing to share her dream stories with the world so other men and women may be saved by them. So, these are Mary's dreams.

About three years ago, I got an intuitive insight dream telling me that if I did not leave my unhappy marriage, I would get breast cancer. The recurrent dreams felt so vivid and were often followed by day visions. My intuitive dreams were always the same—short, to the point, and often happened when I first fell asleep or as early morning dreams.

A Few Days to Live Dream

In the intuitive dreams/nightmares, I had lost all my hair and looked very thin and frail. I looked like I only had a few days to live, which scared me.

Somehow, I managed to forget about the dreams and carried on with my busy life. A year later, I started feeling a lump in my left breast. It was very alarming. After going to the doctor to have it checked out, the doctor said it was nothing to be concerned about, which to me felt like the checkup was not enough. I wanted him to do more tests.

The Dark Mass

Over the next few months, my left breast felt like it was being taken over by something. The best way to describe this feeling is to say "the energy felt off." After I contacted my doctor, an ultrasound/mammogram was performed and my physician found a dark mass.

That is when I thought, *OMG! Here we go!* Memories of dream and nightmares followed by visions came back. I felt so alarmed, I ended up having a consultation with Mona Lisa Schulz, a Hay House medical intuitive. One of the first things she said was, "I see some energy in your left breast. If you don't stop over-caring for people in your life, you will get breast cancer."

Wow! I thought. *Okay. I need to make changes in my life.* And so, I did.

Because of my mental health and wellness-oriented business, people chronically in emotional need are attracted to me. To become aware of "over-caring" for others, my body developed a "warning bell," in the form of feelings of inner irritation. Validation comes from asking myself, *Do you feel dragged down, drained, or over-engaged?* Emotional boundaries became an essential part of my life, and I learned the power of saying no. Self-care, diet, happy thoughts, exercise, and divorce proceedings became my focus.

The next time I went for testing, the dark mass had disappeared, melted away. My dramatic life changes had made it disappear! The power of intuition and dreams... Ya gotta love it!

KAT'S INTERPRETATION

If these were my dreams I would also consider them an "intuitive hit," as Mary did, which is another way of saying a literal precognitive warning dream, because the dream is literal in detail and the message is crystal clear but it all takes place before symptoms in the future. Like many of the dreamers in this book, including myself, Mary's dreams were also recurrent, with accompanying day visions. Her dreams were a very dark, precognitive, call-to-action warning of a future condition. What makes Mary's dream so profound is the dream was validated in the waking world by a medical report but by immediately changing her life, she healed her future.

The "dark mass" disappeared, and the change was verified by more medical tests. Acting on a precognitive dream can alter your life's ending.

DR. BURK'S COMMENTARY

The reading that Mary had from Mona Lisa Schulz, MD, PhD, is also important as it reinforces the theme of the earth element imbalance of over-caring for others described in the stories Amparo and Sunni earlier. Dr. Schulz is the only medical intuitive I know who is also a psychiatrist and neuroscientist, so combining Mary's own intuitive abilities with hers makes for a compelling combination. Good medical intuitives often serve us best when they cause us to believe what our own intuition has already told us, but we want to deny.

PART THREE

*True Dream Stories of
Other Types of Cancers*

And just as the eye bears witness to the peculiar and spontaneous creative activity of living matter, the primordial image expresses the intrinsic and unconditioned creative power of the psyche.
— CARL JUNG, *CW 6, Para 748*

These are stories of people saved by cancer dreams who were not in Dr. Larry Burk's Breast Cancer Dream Project, but who found us through social media or the International Association for the Study of Dreams workshops and talks we did together and alone.

Basal Cell Carcinoma: Medical Introduction

B asal cell carcinoma is the most common skin cancer, with over 4 million cases diagnosed in the United States each year. This type of cancer often develops from precancerous actinic keratoses, which are highly correlated with ultraviolet sun exposure. It rarely metastasizes, so is not life threatening. However, it can be disfiguring and require aggressive MOHS surgery.

Basal cell carcinoma is usually detected by self-examination, prompting a visit to the dermatologist, although it may be overlooked in difficult to visualize areas of the body like the back or inner surface of the ear as described below by Lorraine. Fortunately, she was guided to find her basal cell carcinoma by a persistent dream voice that would wake her up in the morning.

16

The Awakening

Lorraine

My dream was more like an awakening every morning, for at least a year, with this thought in my mind: *there is something in my ear that needs to come out.* The "something" was pea size and appeared to be a ball of wax. However, it produced a spot of blood on the towel after my shower, then turned into a scab. I spoke with my doctor about it and remember saying, "I've got one of those famous 'sores that will not heal.'"

My doctor treated the scab with cryotherapy. My concern was that when the scab was toweled off after my next shower, the cryotherapy would come off with it. I was right. However, before reporting back to the doctor, I suffered a painful bout of bursitis in my neck and shoulder, followed by a back injury from an accident. The two incidents demanded all my focus to heal.

In the meantime, I watched YouTube videos of people getting ear wax removed by undergoing something called ear candling. I was obsessed with ear wax and bought mineral oil from the drugstore to try homegrown remedies. I avoided my doctor because I already felt like a hypochondriac.

After months of pain and medications for my back injury, the subject of my ear was again brought up to my doctor. A biopsy was performed. Unfortunately, my "ear wax" was a basal cell carcinoma. The good news, as told to me, was that if I had to get cancer, this was a good kind to get, because it was self-contained and would not spread. The bad news was that it had grown much larger than the size of a pea.

An appointment was immediately booked for me to see a plastic surgeon, who performed surgery at the local hospital while I was under general anesthetic. This included skin grafting of a skin flap. Weeks later, lab results showed that the plastic surgeon had not gotten all of the cancer, so another operation was scheduled. My end result was having even less of an ear than the first time. However, my ear was saved, and the cancer was gone.

This was three years ago, and my ear still feels stiff and frozen, an alien entity attached to my head. There must be nerve damage, but I'm lucky that is all I have. My younger sister died of cancer at the age of 60. I am grateful to be alive and wish I had recognized the power of my inner voice and reported back to my doctor sooner.

17

My Dream Voice

Angelika Hartmann

Angelika Hartmann from Virginia Beach works in the
holistic wellness field and also heard a dream voice warning
her of a basal cell carcinoma. This is her dream story.

I have had intense dreams since the age of 10. Many are symbolic; some have transitioned loved ones visiting and comforting me. Some dreams foretell future events. Forty-two years in Virginia was always a problem for my fair skin, and I had problems in the summertime with rashes and breakouts. That is why it took two years of dealing with a persistent rash the size of a dime on my nose to be correctly diagnosed as basal cell carcinoma. I did see several doctors, who told me not to worry.

In one of my dreams my subconscious voice told me: *You have skin cancer.* I felt it to be correct and made an appointment with a dermatologist to be biopsied. Cancer was confirmed and removed in 2016. I am still under observation. My prognosis is good, but all my companions worship the outdoors, and they have to deal with me not being outdoors for fun before 6 p.m.

18

Saving Face

Dana Walden

For months I had been fatigued. Before going to sleep one night during the worst of it, I prayed for a dream to shed some light. Here is the dream I received.

The Worm and the Bird Dream

There is a clearing/meadow surrounded by a forest with a snow-capped mountain to the north. The sun is warm. The grass is cool. A few puffy white clouds are scattered throughout the sky. The wind is silent. There is a small clear stream cutting through the edge of the meadow.

An antelope sits at the north edge of the field, a wolf at the south, a bear at the west, and a deer at the east. A bluebird flies back and forth between the wolf and antelope, resting a short time on both.

I lay down face up in the middle of the meadow. An eagle is circling. I have the sense it's sealing the ring, as all the unseen animals in the forest are singing their prayers for me. The sun warms me as a shaman appears to tell me the sun belongs to the Indians, who are the caretakers of the earth. They have joined in the healing.

The bluebird flies to me and sits on my stomach, then runs up and down both legs. She begins to peck on the left side of my nose next to my left eye, grabs a worm from the hole, and starts to pull it out.

I feel the worm go deep and wrap around my spine. I lie and wait for the bluebird to take the worm all the way out but worry the bird will eat the disease. A "knowing" states my disease will be transformed into food to feed the bluebird family for generations—a gift for helping in the healing.

The bluebird pulls the longest worm I've ever seen all the way out of the side of my nose, and, with the worm in tow, it flies away.

There's a hole left between my eye and nose, but the eagle swoops down and shits in the wound. Somehow, I know this is good luck and good for me, as it seals the hole. The four animals: wolf, bear, antelope, deer rotate around the meadow; each sits at the different directions until they all come back to their original places. At that time, I'm told these are my animals, this is my sacred meadow, and to mark my spot in the center, where I am.

I awaken feeling so blessed and grateful. Later that morning, when shaving, I noticed a mole I hadn't ever seen before between my eye and the left side of my nose. *That's weird,* I thought.

I'm normally not one to quickly go to the doctor's, even when the writing has been on the wall for years. But in this moment my dream flashes back to me, especially the part about the bird pulling out the long worm. I knew I had to go get it checked out.

A few days later an appointment is made with a dermatologist. After looking at the spot on my face, he said, "What has taken you so long to get in here?"

Following a biopsy, the pathology report stated it was an aggressive basal cell cancer. My doctor insisted on doing immediate surgery on the worm-like cancer in my face! Fortunately, he was a big Beverly Hills plastic surgeon, so I have no scar.

The surgery was successful, and the doctor praised me for coming in when I did, or it would have required much more extensive surgery. In case you're wondering, I was sent home with a hole in my face, just like in my dream, but it was covered with a surgical Band-Aid instead of bird shit. I'm forever grateful for that dream, which helped me to not only save face (pun intended), and maybe even my brain, but also connected me with some very powerful animal guides, which have since become part of my meditation and lead me to a place of empowerment, peace, and deep ease (instead of dis-ease).

KAT'S INTERPRETATION

If Dana's dream were mine, I would call it a diagnostic and symbolic healing dream with shades of a shamanic dream; a dream journey in which the dreamer often goes to new places in order to access knowledge, meet power animals as healing guides, and find power plants. I would consider it diagnostic, because it shows the dreamer a worm in his face eating its way to his spine, which diagnosis a problem. It is healing because it is filled with *totem animals* surrounding him while he is grounded in a *sacred meadow* of healing. The *bluebird* appears to be "checking him out," up and down, before latching onto the worm. Bluebirds are considered a sign of optimism in a dream. A *wolf* in a dream can be seen as sacred wisdom. A *bear* may be symbolic of a highly protective inner-mother, protecting she-bear. In many cases, the bear may represent a meeting with dangerous emotions and overcoming them, often with unconditional love.

When an *antelope* visits your dreams, it may symbolize the ability to achieve whatever you want, including your dreams, as long as you put forth the time and effort. Antelopes were often considered the first magical and mystical unicorns, because their profile looked like a single, long, thin horn protruding from their forehead. A *deer* in a dream may be a positive symbol of the gentle, spiritually awakening aspect of your life. Dana's totem animals stand at the spots indicating the four directions. They then create a Healing Circle of Life by rotating clockwise (forward in time) through all four directional points until they return to their original position on the Compass of Life.

The message I might take from the dream is the totem animals foretold of health and healing in the future. I am so glad Dana went home with nothing in the hole in his face, including cancer. However, in American Indian folklore, dreaming of a bird pooping on you is a sign of luck. The amount of luck present in any particular poo seems to be influenced by the type of bird doing the pooping. In Dana's dream, it is an eagle. I would consider the hole in my face being filled with eagle poo a healthy and lucky omen.

Like many of the other dreamers shared in this book, Lorraine and Angelika heard a voice. If these were my dreams, I would call them auditory diagnostic dreams often described as an awake dream; on the threshold of consciousness during the time of entering or exiting a dream, known as a hypnagogic state of consciousness. A waking dream may be a type of a lucid dream that may contain lucid thought. Lorraine and Angelika heard distinct words rather than saw signs or symbols. Early-morning dreams are thought to be the easiest to remember because they happen so close to waking up. Their dreams were validated by pathology reports.

DR. BURK'S COMMENTARY

Basal cell carcinoma may present as a suspicious mole like Dana's, or a sore that won't heal like Lorraine's, or as a rash that persists like Angelika's. Precancerous skin lesions are so common that it may take a while for the significance of a particular skin cancer to become visible. Dana's worm imagery is a good metaphor for the more aggressive infiltrative kind of basal cell carcinoma, as it may invade along nerves going deeper into the skin in a worm-like fashion. In the other two examples, it was a dream voice without explicit imagery that provided the necessary motivation to persist in seeking the eventual diagnosis. Even though these cancers don't metastasize, early detection is still important to avoid disfigurement.

Benign and Malignant Brain Tumors: Medical Introduction

(Featuring Mark Ruffalo's Dream Cancer Story)

B rain tumors are one of the most frightening types of cancer due to the poor prognosis and the severe associated disability. Also concerning is the fact that the incidence of malignant cancers such as glioblastoma multiforme has increased by 39 percent since the 1970s. Because these tumors are still relatively rare, there is no cost-effective screening method for detection.

Actor Mark Ruffalo had a dream about having a brain tumor in 2001, which proved to be an accurate prediction, but fortunately, it turned out to be a benign acoustic neuroma.[54] He described that "It was like no other dream I'd ever had."

In his own words to his doctor from previously published interviews: "Listen, I really had a scary dream last night, and you'll probably think I'm crazy, but, um... but I think I have a brain tumor, and I would really like to get it, uh... checked out. The impression from the dream was that "It had to be dealt with immediately."

To reassure him the doctor ordered CT and MRI scans, which led to the diagnosis of a golf ball-sized tumor near his ear, much to the shock of the physician. Ruffalo noted that he "didn't have any displayed symptoms" and pre-operative testing showed that he had only a 7 percent hearing loss in that ear compared with the other, which "was undiscernible to me." After successful surgery that sacrificed the nerve to his ear, and a lengthy recovery, he resumed his acting career, with a complete hearing loss on that side being the only major residual effect.

19

Into the Panther's Cage

Deb Dutilh

Kat met Deb Dutilh when Kat was presenting at an IASD conference. Deb was also blessed with a series of warning, diagnostic, and precognitive dreams as described in her story below, and which she has performed as a one-woman theatrical show, Into the Panther's Cage. She is lucky to still be alive after treatment for the dreaded glioblastoma multiforme warned about in her dreams, shortly after her ex-husband died of the same cancer. Here are excerpts from her dream diary, beginning with the initial discovery of her ex-husband's brain tumor.

The call from my son Guillaume came on September 15, 2009. He was visiting his dad, my ex-husband, Jean-François, in France. After trying to work through his sudden bizarre behavior, we had divorced after 27 years of marriage. We still cared deeply about each other and promised to always be there for one another.

Jean-Francois died shortly after the phone call from my son, from glioblastoma multiforme, or GBM, a deadly brain tumor.

A Visit from Jean-François: Walking in His Shoes

I'm dreaming that Jean-François gives me a picture of a playful seal he's drawn. We're walking hand in hand along the beach, and I'm wearing his worn leather hiking boots with their thick, sturdy soles and the long red laces wound around my ankles a few times. Then suddenly, we're inside a big store like Target, driving his car up and down the aisles, looking for an exit.

I wake up feeling anxious and not liking the meaning of this dream at all! I know the seal represents our pact of always being connected through our kids. Does walking in his shoes mean I have a deadly health issue like he had, too? Do those thick, sturdy soles and long red shoelaces symbolize our forever entwined souls? What does the future hold in store for me? Will I need to be shopping around for solutions? Will I be exiting this world anytime soon, the way he did?

Not wanting to believe what my intuition is telling me and the obvious metaphors, I try to brush my concerns aside. But my fear is lurking. My health is normal, but this dream isn't. Will any symptoms appear?

Ironically, four years to the day after Jean-François had his grand mal seizure, I got the big symptom: an excruciating migraine that landed me in urgent care.

The doctor reassured me that headaches could have many causes and 99 percent of the time; without other significant symptoms, they are not a source of concern. My bloodwork looked good, and I was functioning normally, although very dehydrated from the vomiting.

I was sent home with pain pills, told to drink lots of fluids, rest, and return in a week or so for a follow up. It sounded like treatment for a common cold without chicken soup!

And then, my intuition kicked in. *I'm not buying this simple diagnosis! The absence of symptoms didn't mean the absence of disease.*

My Life Celebration: Blackbird Dream

I'm at a big party with my favorite music playing "Blackbird" by Paul McCartney. Everyone is talking about me—a lot—about how courageous I WAS! I try to capture people's attention, but nobody sees or hears me! "Oh, my God! I'm at my own life celebration! Everyone is here celebrating my life! This has to be a dream!" I sit up in bed and raise my arm in front of my face, yelling and trying to stop the onslaught of anecdotes and memories of my life.

Finally, I awaken, shaken up from this dream. The dream confirms something is terribly wrong with me and can kill me if action isn't taken *now*.

My doctor listened intently as I told him about the recent dreams and what my intuition was telling me. The irony of the dates lining up disturbed me, too. My sons had already lost their dad to a brain tumor. No one deserves this experience once, let alone twice! I could not bear seeing that fear in their eyes or hearing it in their voices. We all needed peace of mind.

Fortunately, my doctor agreed there might be something to my dreams and referred me to a neurologist for an MRI to rule out anything serious.

Still, at this point, I was functioning correctly, and my only symptoms were three migraines and frightening prophetic dreams. The neurologist was not overly concerned and handed me a chart to note down all the details about my headaches. This was a useless exercise. If we were leaving no stone unturned, let's look under the biggest boulders first.

"Doctor, if we were talking about your wife or daughter, and regardless of the cost, would you do an MRI?"

"Yes, I would," he replied.

On the morning of October 30, without telling anyone, I calmly went for the MRI. As I prepared to leave, the technician stops me.

"Deborah, we've found something we're concerned about. I need to take you to the emergency room."

"We Found Something"

Since no one is letting me out of their sights, I assume I too have a brain tumor. In the ER, expecting the worst, I had my brief pity party; cursing the world, the gods and, whoever could hear me!

At that moment, I make my decision. Whatever the diagnosis, prognosis, and statistics, I have only one thing to say to the world. "Watch me beat you!"

On November 2, 2013, Jean-François' 60th birthday, the apricot-sized tumor was completely removed. I was released from the hospital two days later, on *my* 60th birthday. Clearly, this wasn't the birthday gift, celebration, or trendy asymmetrical haircut I had planned!

It turns out that I'm now admitted into the PhD program at the Academy of Brain Tumors with a glioblastoma multiforme, the most common, deadliest, and highest-grade brain tumor! I'm a smart cookie. Oh, the irony of it all! I would have been content with a low to average grade. I am stunned by the confirmation that my dreams were right and that the visit from Jean-François saved my life with early detection. How do our departed loved ones know these things when we don't?

To help me heal, I start writing my solo performance to share my story.

Into the Panther's Cage Dream

Before falling asleep, I ask my totem animal for guidance and confirmation. I need to know that sharing my story on stage will inspire people.

I'm hiking along a parched riverbed. Black Panther silently slinks up behind me. A man appears and orders her into a cave that has appeared in the hillside. Bars drop and cage her in. Next, he orders her to guard this dry riverbed before disappearing. I must release her, but how?

My English teacher skills come to the rescue, reminding me that prepositions are taught in pairs of opposites. Knowing you can't get out of something you haven't gotten yourself into, I realize the only way to free her is to get into the cage with her.

Slipping easily through the bars, completely trusting her as my guardian,
I snuggle up to her luxurious silky chest, feeling it gently rise as I relax in sync
with her warm, calm breathing.

Suddenly with a whisper of air, the bars disappear. Black Panther and
I descend the dusty trail into an abundant green jungle leading to a natural
amphitheater filled to capacity. She leads me to front and center stage before
taking a regal pose beside me.

When the music starts, the crowd rises to join me in song and dance.

I wake up elated knowing she has confirmed my calling of sharing my story. Stepping into the Panther's Cage proved I could courageously face my greatest fears and survive. I also created the void within me for Black Panther spirit to return, to reclaim her power and replenish my own soul's dried up riverbed of creativity.

Today, with Black Panther faithfully by my side and no evidence of disease, I share my surreal journey of dreams, resilience, and humor on stage to inspire and give hope to others also striking back at life's curve balls.

It's been three and a half years since my diagnosis with GBM, and six since Jean-François died. He still visits me in dreams, taking me to his world and reassuring me that it is not my time yet. I am blessed with proof that love prevails, and that I have a guardian angel watching over me.

KAT'S INTERPRETATION

Deb is fantastic at understanding her dreams. If these were my dreams I would call the first one a diagnostic dream and visitation filled with symbolism; a visit from her dead husband putting his boots on her feet on the *beach*, which can be seen as an area that separates two land masses or two states of being: the living and the dead. *His boots on her feet* may symbolize the saying: "Walk a mile in my shoes." Into the Panther's Cage is an example of an Incubated Dream, because Deb set her dream intention before sleep and saw the answer. Animals in dreams are valuable and unique to the dreamer. Deb saw *walking into the cage of the Black Panther* as facing her darkest fear. And *attending your own "life celebration"* might be interpreted as another phrase for a funeral-wake, which speaks volumes to the urgency of seeking help. Deb's diagnostic dreams used symbolism and conversations to show the near future if she ignored them. Her dreams were validated by pathology reports. Her precognitive dream of performing before an audience has become a reality.

DR. BURK'S COMMENTARY

Actor Mark Ruffalo's dream warning is an exception to many of the other dream stories in the book, in that his tumor was benign but still had life-threatening implications. He had the same sense of the profound urgency of the dream shared by many of the breast cancer dreamers, and he took the risk of sharing it with his doctor, despite the lack of symptoms. As someone in the public eye, he has also been quite courageous in sharing the dream diagnosis story, which occurred just as his career began to take off.

In Deb Dutilh's first dream, she had a visitation from her deceased husband similar to the dead relatives who visited some of the breast cancer dreamers with warning messages. A family history is a common risk factor in breast cancer, so having a mother or grandmother who died of the same disease show up in the dream state might not be that surprising, considering that breast cancer is a common illness.

Since brain cancer is relatively rare, and after-death dream communications from deceased spouses are relatively common, interpreting the rather vague symbols in the dream as a concrete sign of brain cancer is rather improbable. However, it is understandable that the images of walking in his shoes and looking for an exit could create an ominous feeling upon awakening.

The dream could have been precognitive of the occurrence of the headache less than a month later, but at the time could also have been attributed to lingering stress from the traumatic experience of the dream as a sort of psychosomatic self-fulfilling prophecy. Attending her own memorial in the second dream was reminiscent of the life review that occurs during a classical near-death experience, providing timely clarification of the first dream and encouraging her to go for the MRI and surgery. Perhaps our deceased family members do sometimes act as guardian dream angels delivering timely warning messages.

Colon Cancer:
Medical Introduction

Colon cancer is the second leading cause of cancer death in the United States, and 4 percent of people are diagnosed with colorectal cancer during their lifetimes. The risk goes up with a family history or a personal history of polyps. The risk increases with age, so recommendations for screening begin at age 50, with colonoscopy every 10 years, barium enema every five years, or fecal occult blood tests yearly.

Colon cancer can be hard to detect in its early stages, as the symptoms may be nonspecific. Since it is such a common cancer, it is not surprising that there would be reports of colon cancer dreams. After my breast cancer dreams paper came out, I discovered that one of my high school classmates had a personal story about having a life-saving colon cancer dream. For the purposes of this book, we are using the name Aislinn by request, not her real name.

20

The Bloody Toilet

Aislinn

This is my story regarding my dream (or nightmare, if you will) of colon cancer. I was a busy mother of two teenagers in the spring of 2003 and working part-time for my husband, teaching a theater class, and serving on two volunteer boards.

Happily married, and blessed with a beautiful and active life, I felt terrific. I hit the gym three times a week, walked, swam, and went on ski trips with my family. I saw my PCP (primary care physician) once a year and did everything he asked me to do: bloodwork, mammograms, Pap smears, and so on.

My eating habits were healthy, preferring fish, chicken, fruits, and vegetables. Sweets were enjoyed sparingly. My mother was an organic cook, so she instilled healthy eating habits that I continue to this day. I had no fatigue or incidences of rectal bleeding.

As time went on, I became sensitive to fried foods and fresh cream. Stomach pains would make me run to the bathroom with diarrhea. There was occasional constipation. Since these incidents were not chronic, I made a mental note to talk to my PCP about possible irritable bowel syndrome and went on my merry way. Then I started having recurring dreams.

The Bloody Toilet Dream

Entering a stark white bathroom, I look into a commode, which was filled with bright red blood. It was horrifying!

This happened a few times, which was a red flag to me, but I did not reveal these dreams to my PCP. I did not want him to think I was crazy or unstable, so I just stuck to the facts. On some subconscious level I knew I was ill.

The Colonoscopy

My PCP listened to me and recommended a colonoscopy, as I was nearing the age when this test is recommended. I had a tumor the size of a pea and had a re-section of my colon. Nine lymph nodes were removed—of the nine, two nodes were positive for cancer cells. So my oncologist recommended adjuvant chemotherapy. The chemo did not make me suffer as many do with vicious nausea. I considered myself very, very fortunate.

That was nearly 13 years ago, and my health has been good, thank God. I exercise, take meditation classes from a Buddhist monk, watch my diet, keep my health appointments, and have moved forward in a positive way.

I learned it is important to listen to yourself. Dreams are an indication of what is going on in your life. My story is shared often, as I am an open and honest person. I feel that if it helps one individual, my life would be complete.

21

Feces Everywhere!

Aisha Umar

A year later, in 2016, Dr. Larry Burk was contacted by Aisha Umar,
a Muslim woman from Canada who started to have colon cancer-related
dreams five years prior to her diagnosis. Her story is a cautionary one,
as it shows that very disturbing dreams can be too embarrassing to
share with your doctor, resulting in a life-threatening delay in taking
action on them.

My name is Aisha Umar. Several years ago, my dreams began about feces being everywhere, and, in 2015, I was diagnosed with stage 4 colon cancer, even though my illness had no symptoms.

Here is my story.

I've always been very healthy and took my health for granted. But I have had my share of stressors. At the age of 35, my painful custody battle and divorce began, which lasted several years. At this time, anxiety issues began to emerge, and at age 40, I went through a year of severe depression.

It was just prior to this depression (and during it) that I experienced non-stop dreams and visions (while I was awake) of feces.

Feces Everywhere Dream

There was no blood in the stool, but I kept seeing piles of my feces in inappropriate places. It was so consuming I couldn't stop thinking about it (and I didn't share it with anyone, because it sounded ludicrous). I was raised a Muslim, and I kept seeing my feces on the Quran (which would really upset me and I'd plead with God to make me stop having this vision). Anyway, it was constantly in my mind: I would be having this vision of feces on my desk, on religious books, being thrown at me, while I was having meetings at work, sitting with my daughter, sleeping. It was to the point where I was in tears and could not distract myself from having this vision.

Eventually, the nightmare went away.

A Diagnosis and Two Surgeries

At 45, I was diagnosed with stage 4 colon cancer, resulting in two surgeries and eight chemo sessions. The doctors are hopeful (but we are really in a wait-and-see situation). The first surgery was colon and liver, and the colon has been okay since then. A year later, the second surgery, of the liver, was also successful. The doctors say colon is one of the few stage 4 cancers that can be cured, but as you know, there are no guarantees. My determination to fight is the direct result of my love for my 16-year-old daughter.

The colon surgeons believe cancer started in my system in my late 30s, the same time these visions started. Making that connection would never have occurred to me, because we do not have a history of cancer in our family, and truthfully, I do not know much about colon cancer. And the dreams were so embarrassing to me that talking about them with my general practitioner (GP) would have been impossible. I thought I was insane. What would he think? It was only after my diagnosis that it became apparent to me that there had to be a connection, because the visions were nonstop, constant, so vivid, and to the point.

I was constantly in tears. I struggled with the uncertainty of it all but believed my body was trying to tell me something. Sadly, I was too embarrassed by it to do anything about it. Instead, if I had thought that maybe something was wrong with my bowel movements and what disease might be associated with that, I might have gotten the right answer. Hindsight.

I am recovering from the surgery and going back to work soon, and I try to make peace with the situation. It is my hope that my story helps other people. If it had not happened to me, I would not have believed it.

KAT'S INTERPRETATION

If Aislinn's dream were mine, I would call it a recurrent diagnostic dream/nightmare that uses literal symbolism as a call to action. Fear from a nightmare is a great motivator to remember the dream contents and do something about it to make it stop recurring. If Aisha's dream were mine, I might wonder if it may have been a precognitive dream showing what may happen in the future, since the dream may have been just before the illness began to grow. It may also be a dream duality, describing both Aisha Umar's daily life and physical health.

As many of the other dreamers in this book have pointed out, myself included, many diagnostic health-related dream messages recur until they drive the dreamer to distraction, or the doctor.

They are experienced in the waking world as well as the dream world. As Aisha Umar stated, in a play on words, *hindsight*—looking at her back end was likely the key to the solution of her "crappy" problem. We are glad she moved past her shame to share her story with us.

DR. BURK'S COMMENTARY

The dreams of blood in the toilet and feces in inappropriate places certainly draw attention to the colon in a dramatic way; however, there was no specific mention of cancer in either dream narrative, so other types of interpretations are possible. The blood could have also represented hemorrhage from another source in the colon, such as colitis, severe hemorrhoids, an anal fissure, or an abnormal blood vessel, in a condition known as angiodysplasia. It could also have been blood in the urine from a kidney problem.

The possibility of a metaphor should also be considered, particularly regarding the fecal material. In the context of a painful divorce, those kinds of dream images might not be surprising. The colon is one of our primary organs of elimination, so the desire to let go of a "crappy" marriage could manifest through the subconscious as a response to overwhelming stress. The five-year interval also raises the question of how long it could take a persistent metaphor to turn into a real physical problem.

When I made my first presentation on cancer dreams, in 2013, one of the members of the International Society for the Study of Dreams mentioned that she had a client with vivid dreams of having cancer in the groin. After all the radiology studies turned out to be negative, she concluded it must be a metaphor. Then she realized that her boyfriend was a Cancer astrological sign and was behaving malignantly, so she dumped him. If she had ignored the dream warning and married him instead, I wonder if she would have eventually manifested a tumor there.

Lung Cancer:
Medical Introduction

Lung cancer deaths every year are greater in number than from breast, colon, and prostate cancers combined. It is the leading cause of cancer-related death in both men and women, and accounts for 14 percent of new cancer cases in the United States. Cigarette smoking increases the risk of lung cancer by 13 times in women, and by 23 times in men.

Annual screening for lung cancer with low-dose computed tomography is recommended for adults aged 55 to 80 years who have a 30 pack-a-year smoking history and currently smoke or have quit within the past 15 years. My friend Carl O. Helvie, the host of the *Holistic Health Show* and president of The Carl O Helvie Holistic Cancer Foundation, is still alive over 40 years after his dream diagnosis of lung cancer, as he recounts in this excerpt from his book.[55]

22

"Go For An X-ray!"

Carl O. Helvie, RN, DrPH

I am a registered nurse with a doctorate in public health and wellness, so I am well grounded in public health, nursing, and holistic health. At the time of my diagnosis, I had completed my doctorate in public health at Johns Hopkins University and was teaching graduate and undergraduate nursing students and public health students at a local university. *In July 1974, I awoke from a dream telling me to go for a chest X-ray.*

I have learned to listen to my dreams because they have often guided me on health matters, in problem solving, and with finding things. I thus tell friends that when God speaks, I listen. When I contacted my physician and asked for a referral for an X-ray, he asked if I had symptoms. I told him no but insisted on a referral, and he sent me for X-rays. As a conservative, traditional physician, he would not have understood about the guidance offered in dreams, and I did not mention it. But I was persistent in my request for an X-ray.

The Spot

After receiving the X-ray report, my physician called and asked me to come to his office. There, he told me that they had found a spot on my lungs that had not been there six months earlier and requested I go into the hospital for a biopsy. Following the lung biopsy, and while I was still in the hospital, my physician reported that it was a malignant tumor and that I needed immediate surgery. He had also arranged for a surgeon to speak with me. I told both doctors I was not willing to rush into any decision about surgery but wanted all of the information available, so I could go home, pray, think about it, and make a rational decision. He told me I would be dead in six months without immediate surgery and repeated this several times.

Alternative Holistic Treatments

I reminded him that the decision about surgery and the responsibility for my life was mine, and his responsibility was to give me the information available to help me make a decision. Despite my background, or maybe because of it, I found the diagnosis of six months to live and the prospects of being disabled for that period as a result of using conventional treatment frightening. Thus, my selection was alternative holistic treatments to deal with my lung cancer. For the 39 years since then, to date I have remained cancer-free, which is relatively unusual with traditional care.

KAT'S INTERPRETATION

I agree with Dr. Burk that no dream interpretation is necessary other than to say this was an audio diagnostic dream validated by a pathology report. But I want to share with you the importance of embracing inner guidance and synchronicities when they appear in life, because they are what I call "God winks," reassurance that you are on the right path, which Carl was, and ultimately saved his life after being told he had only six months to live.

I met Dr. Carl O. Helvie on the social media site LinkedIn, when he asked if he could be my guest on *The Kat Kanavos Show* on internet TV and invited me to be on his internet radio show. This was before Dr. Larry Burk and I had decided to write this book on the Breast Cancer Dream Project. I was unaware that Larry and Carl knew each other. Since that time, I have discovered that Carl studied dream interpretation and therapy 41 years ago with Dr. Ursula Martens-Jahoda who, according to Carl, "was in my study group and offered to work with me by studying her dreams which helped me make a decision based upon spiritual guidance. We all agreed that treating the disease naturally was the best approach."

Dr. Ursula Martens-Jahoda, now deceased, was an instructor, owner, director of the Physical Research and Development Foundation and Academy in Virginia Beach, and my dream mentor when I was diagnosed with breast cancer all three times. Ursula's family had been close friends with Edgar Cayce known as "The Sleeping Prophet" and she showed me pictures of her as a young girl sitting on Edgar Cayce's lap. In 1990, I had attended the academy with my husband, and Ursula and I became close friends. I wrote about working through my dreams with her in my book *Surviving Cancerland*, for which she wrote an endorsement. To add to these amazing circumstances, pediatrician Dr. Kathi Kemper, whose stories are also in this book, was Dr. Ursula Martens-Jahoda's "adopted daughter." We were introduced by Ursula, and I was invited to Kathi's Chinese New Year party in Boston during my treatment. We are still close friends who feel more like family.

We (Dr. Larry Burk, Dr. Kathi Kemper, Dr. Ursula Martens-Jahoda, Dr. Carl Helvie, and I) have all come together, unplanned, decades later, through the validation and importance of dreams in this book. Like John Lennon sang, *Come Together, Right Now...* over dreams. Wink, wink.

DR. BURK'S COMMENTARY

Carl's dream does not require interpretation, as he was fortunate to get direct guidance to go for a diagnostic test. Carolyn Kinney and others have received similar accurate information upon waking that led them to take action, sometimes including a voice command. Carl was already an experienced dreamer who had learned to trust in such divine guidance.

Melanoma Dreams:
Medical Introduction

M elanoma accounts for less than 1 percent of all skin cancer cases, but most of the deaths. Risk factors for melanoma include fair skin, multiple moles, repeated sunburns, and a family history. There are specific guidelines that provide criteria for evaluating whether a mole needs to be biopsied or not. Prognosis is tied closely to early detection through self-examination, so paying attention to any suspicious skin lesions is important. Dreams may also prompt evaluation by a physician, as noted by both Diane Powell, MD, and Linda Ellerker below.

23

The "What If?" Nightmare

Diane Powell, MD

Several years ago, I awoke in a panic from a nightmare. I did not remember the nightmare, but the first thought I had upon awakening was, *What if it is melanoma?* I'm not prone to nightmares and was not worried about the new mole on the back of my leg. It looked perfectly healthy. I had no history of sunburns. In fact, I never spent much time in the sun and barely remember having had tans.

"It's Not Melanoma; It Is Melanoma. It's Not..."

No one in my family had ever had melanoma. Still, I showed it to my then-husband, an oncologist.

"That's not melanoma," he said, looking at my leg. "It's perfectly round, has a uniform color, and is less than a half centimeter."

"I know," I said, feeling almost foolish for asking. "I went to the same medical school as you. It's just unusual for me to wake up terrorized."

But What If?

I did not think about it again, that is until I awoke the following month in a panic. *But what if it is melanoma?* I sought reassurance from my husband a second time. After the third awakening, I scheduled an appointment.

The Appointment

"It's not melanoma," said my internist, with certainty. "But if you want me to take it off, I will."

"Please do," I said. "At least it will help me sleep better."

I returned the following week to have the sutures removed and to receive the pathology report. My internist looked her usual serene self, so I immediately felt relieved. Upon opening my chart, her expression changed to concern.

"Oh, I'm sorry. I didn't review this before you arrived. It *is* melanoma. Fortunately, it is in situ and can be cured by a wider excision. Good thing we caught it early."

24

The House with Bloody Walls

Linda Ellerker

A prophetic dream about my cancer saved my life! I don't usually remember dreams, nor did I pay much attention to my dreams at that time. This was 20 years ago.

> In my dream, I went into a construction site where homes were under construction. I went into the first house, looked around, then came back out. I then went into the second house, looked around, then came back out. When I moved into the third house, there was blood all over the walls.

I woke up with a feeling of dread and couldn't shake the dream. At that time, I was feeling really good, no problems at all, except my doctor of Chinese medicine had taken my pulses during a checkup and told me my life energy was low. Having no idea what that meant because I was feeling so good, an appointment was made with my medical doctor who performed a physical. He told me my health was perfect.

It Kept Bugging Me

Still, the dream haunted me. I noticed a mole on the back of my neck and thought about the construction site in my dream. The doctor and the dermatologist both insisted it looked fine. I insisted on a biopsy because of the dream. It was precancerous. I thought, "House No. 1." A while later, I noticed a mole on my shoulder: House No. 2. It was precancerous.

Almost a year went by, and the dream began to haunt me again. It kept bugging me, and I could see nothing on my body except the scar from the last biopsy that didn't look right to me.

When I talked to the doctor, he said it was just scar tissue. I asked for a referral to a dermatologist. The dermatologist looked at the scar and said it looked just fine and did not want to do a biopsy as it would make the scar bigger.

Of course, this is news everyone wants to hear. "Do not worry, everything is just fine."

The Third House

The dream, however, made me insist things were not fine. This was the third house, and things were not fine on this building site. The doctor reluctantly took the biopsy, and it came back with the diagnosis of melanoma.

If it had not been for the dream, I would not have insisted on doing the biopsy and left the appointment thinking all was okay. I immediately began working with several alternative practitioners, including acupuncture, herbals, diet, supplements, and energy practices such as reiki and tai chi.

Confidence from a Dream

The dream also gave me the confidence to approach the negative prognosis with the belief that everything was going to be okay, because my body would have warned me in that dream if I were meant to die. Why would the dream insist I seek help if my situation were hopeless?

That was 20 years ago. Since then, I listen to my gut instincts and to my body. I want everyone to know how important it is to listen to their instincts, whether they come through in a dream or some other form of intuition. Don't be afraid to persevere and follow through on what you "know."

KAT'S INTERPRETATION

If Dr. Powell's dream were mine, I'd define it as a recurrent diagnostic waking dream, because she heard Lucid words just as she was waking from her sleep state, known as the hypnagogic state of consciousness, or threshold of consciousness, much like a number of other dreamers in this book. Linda's dream used the symbolism of a *house*, which in the dream world may symbolize our body. If this were my dream, i'd define it as a symbolic precognitive diagnostic dream. It is diagnostic because it showed three different construction sites, of which two had precancer found right away. It is precognitive because the third house (body) had dangerous melanoma that was not identified until it began on an old scar a year later. That was the blood on the walls. Both types of dreams are validated by pathology reports.

Dreams are often as unique as the dreamer and contain the dreamer's particular dream language, as seen here with *three houses*. *Three* is the number that can represent the Holy Trinity of Father, Son, and Holy Ghost, or id, ego, and super-ego, and is also the number often associated with shamanic dreams containing spiritual messages. The different floors of the house were *under construction* which is change or repair. The symbolism made perfect sense to the dreamer. Like many of the dreams in this book, once awake the dream is almost impossible to "shake" or forget until the correct action is taken.

DR. BURK'S COMMENTARY

These two stories provide quite a contrast in dream messages, both triggered by seeing a rather innocuous mole. In Dr. Powell's case, no dream was actually remembered, but a persistent panicky message was received on three different mornings, compelling her to go to the internist for an evaluation despite reassurances that it looked benign. Importantly, the message itself was very specific and came just a week after noticing the mole.

On the other hand, Linda Ellerker's dream was much more nonspecific, requiring her to interpret it in the context of her personal health concerns. Houses can be representative of the body, so having blood on the walls may indicate a problem with the surface covering or skin. Correlating the concept of a construction site with a wound undergoing scarring during repair was very important in this case. Also, the numerical sequence was useful in shifting her attention to the most important third house. It just goes to show that our intuition may be more accurate than even the best clinical judgment based on years of experience.

Ovarian Cancer:
Medical Introduction

Ovarian cancer is the fifth leading cause of cancer-related death in women, and it is the deadliest of reproductive cancers. Overall survival rate at five years is 46 percent, with survival being highly correlated with detection and treatment at an early stage. Since the early disease is often asymptomatic, diagnosis depends on transvaginal ultrasound or the CA125 blood test. Unfortunately, these tests are relatively nonspecific, so screening is usually only considered in women at high risk, with a family history of ovarian or early-onset breast cancer, especially those with the BRCA gene.

Jill Yankee's story below is typical in that she had a family history of ovarian cancer, but also atypical, due to her young age compared to most women who are diagnosed at an older age.

25

The Ugly Doctor

Jill Yankee

I think I was always prepared for ovarian cancer because my mother's sister died of it when she was only 43 years of age. I was four years old at the time, but remember it. My mom warned me, "Jill, you be on the lookout for it, and your sister as well." I think I just always figured "it" was coming.

This dream was several months pre-diagnosis. My husband and I had gone to the beach one day, and that night I had a dream. I'm very fair skinned, so I do think about skin cancer and had thought about it that day.

The Ugly Doctor Dream

In my dream, I went to a doctor. He was going to look me over for skin cancer. I was surprised at how physically ugly the doctor was (this makes sense later). He looked me over and said I did not have any skin cancer, but because he was very thorough, he was going to take blood so he could "look inside to see what was going on." Then the dream changed, and I was on the telephone with the nurse. She told me the results of the blood test. She said, "You have cancer," and as I was waking up, I wondered if it was ovarian cancer or colon cancer.

The reality of the dream came to fruition a few months later. It was ovarian cancer, but it was sitting on the colon. They called a colon specialist into my surgery, in case they needed to take part of the bowel, but fortunately, they did not have to. The surgeon said that the actual cancer mass was a mess, very physically ugly. At first, she thought it was some sort of awful infection, rather than cancer, but the pathology test came back positive. I had more dreams about the cancer before we even knew it was cancer. However, after a pelvic ultrasound, we knew something was going on. I woke up very early one morning in fear. I eventually fell back to sleep and had this dream.

The Spider in the Room

I was in our living room, sitting on the couch with my husband. Everything was white. The walls were white, the ceiling was white, the furniture was white.

I told my husband ,"There's a spider in here. I just know it."

He denied that there was a spider. (He also thought I was being panicky when I had the earlier dream.) He was doing his best to reassure me.

I kept looking up at the ceiling, where the wall meets the ceiling, and kept saying, "I know there's a spider in here. I just know it." But everything was white, and I couldn't see a spider anywhere.

Finally, over my right shoulder, I looked straight up and saw a tiny brown spider descending from the ceiling.

I said, "Aha! There is a spider. I knew it!" But then I thought, "This is not the spider I feared. It's so small and brown, not like the big black spider I thought it would be."

And I almost felt sorry for it and thought maybe I should let it live. But then I knew small spiders get big, and I needed to crush it.

After my diagnosis and surgeries, my oncologist thought it would be best for me to have six chemo treatments because the type of cancer was very aggressive. I was diagnosed with stage 1C ovarian cancer. And, he said the odds of it coming back were too great to take a risk, in his opinion. I did not want chemotherapy, and I had this dream that week.

Something is Hiding In the Boulders

I was looking at a big pile of Bluestone boulders, a kind of rock that is native to the Duluth, Minnesota, area. As I got closer to the pile of stones, I noticed there were spiders in all the crevices and quite a few spiders everywhere on the rocks. We decided to put a kind of sticky tape out on the boulders to catch all the spiders. The next time I looked at the pile of rocks the spiders were gone. This is how I knew I had to have chemotherapy.

KAT'S INTERPRETATION

Jill is another dreamer who has three dreams about the same cancer, and the last dream actually answers her question concerning the use of chemotherapy. Her mind incubated a dream for her answer. If this were my dream, I would define it as an active diagnostic dream that uses symbolism and a play on words, such as a *living room* in her *house*, which could be seen as the place associated with life in the female body, the ovaries. It is also a healing dream because it helps her decide her treatment.

A *brown spider* could possibly be seen as the deadly, tiny, brown recluse spider, whose small bite creates lethal necrosis inside the body, or a brown spider that has not grown to its full black version.

Some dreamers have described cancer as black or as spiders in dreams. As Larry pointed out in his commentary below, spiders are very similar to *crabs*, which are symbolic of cancer. They both belong to the phylum Arthropoda, also known as Euarthropoda, which includes insects and crustaceans. Crabs and spiders are very close cousins, and therefore may share the symbolism of cancer in dreams.

DR. BURK'S COMMENTARY

Jill's family background sensitized her to pay attention to any dream warnings due to a baseline level of anxiety about the possibility of getting this form of cancer; however, her initial dream was triggered by anxiety about skin cancer, instead. The dream was rather accurate in redirecting her to cancers that are associated with an abnormal blood test, most commonly being colon with CEA or ovarian with CA125. It turned out that the cancer was in the ovary sitting on the colon, so the dream message covered both possibilities.

The use of the word "ugly" was precognitive, regarding the surgeon's description of the tumor. The second dream uses the familiar image of a house to represent the body, and white is the typical color of a normal ovary. Spiders, other creepy insects, or crustaceans, such as crabs in Kat's breast cancer dreams, are relatively common symbols that can be interpreted as cancer in the right setting.

Her initial dream occurred when she was asymptomatic, and her cancer was diagnosed still at an early stage, just as it was breaking out of the ovary. Further delay in diagnosis would have worsened the prognosis. Her good outcome may be attributed to the fact that she trusted her intuition, despite her husband's reassurance in the dream and in real life. Plus, her third dream of catching more spiders with sticky tape reinforced the need for chemotherapy and helped her to overcome her objections to it.

Prostate Cancer:
Medical Introduction

But as soon as you take the sexual metaphors as symbols for something
unknown, your conception of the nature of dreams at once deepens.
— **CARL JUNG**, *CW 8, Para 506*

Prostate cancer is the third leading cause of cancer death in men, with 11 percent being diagnosed with it during their lifetimes. Screening has been attempted with a digital rectal examination or PSA blood testing, with mixed results. More cancers may be found using these approaches, but there may be no impact on survival, calling the value of these tests into question.

My friend and colleague Lou Hagood had a series of dreams related to the diagnosis of his prostate cancer, beginning at the 2000 Association for the Study of Dreams (since renamed IASD) conference in Washington, as described below. His description is quite detailed and vivid due to his passion for dream interpretation.[56]

26

The Rape

Lou Hagood

As soon as I closed my eyes, I was bombarded by violent hypnagogic scenes. I knew it would be a rough ride and held on tight. Soon the imagery organized into a dream of running along a path above a beach, arms and legs churning but feet not touching the ground, as if I were flying. A powerful black man pursues me, faster than I, and I know he will catch me. He seizes me from behind and forces me off the trail, down onto the beach toward the water. I struggle but realize my resistance will result in my anal rape there in the sand.

When I returned home to New York from the convention in Washington, I had a number of dying dreams. Our business was in crisis, and our daughter was leaving for freshman year of college, so I considered the dreams symbolic.

Painting Dream

Before our daughter left, I dreamed of walking toward the sunset through a planted field to paint. I am concerned about the men following me, but there is no incident at the end of the field. I turn my back on the sunset and set up my easel facing the field. In Washington, my flight along the beach trail was arrested by the powerful black man, and now my progress toward the sunset is stalked by aggressive men, until I turn my back on the vista to paint. (Both the ungroundedness in Washington and the pursuit of the sunset could be negations of life that have become threatening.)

The black man forced me down to the water, and now I turn my back on the sunset to paint the planted field, correcting my life-negating course. I set up my easel facing not only the planted field but also those dangerous men. (You don't get one without the other.)

The Horns of the Bull

Later that same night I saw myself draped backward between the horns of a bull standing upright on its hind legs. (On the horns of a dilemma, so to speak. The following day, my back went out.)

Before the next Annual Conference of the Association for the Study of Dreams, I was diagnosed with a low-grade prostate cancer, which added a new insight into the Washington dream, with its threatened anal rape and the dying dreams afterward, including the sunset and upright bull dreams just presented. After all, I was draped between the bull's horns backward, balanced on the small of my back, which went out the following day, in the vicinity of my prostate gland.

The prostate gland is in the area of the first chakra as well, which would explain my lack of groundedness as I ran along the beach trail, feet not touching the ground, in the Washington dream. A blockage in the first chakra would correspond with Freud's repressed impulse and Jung's shadow archetype eruption. When my Chinese doctor gave me herbal medication for my blocked chi or vital energy flow, I was reminded of the water that the powerful black person was dragging me down to in the Washington dream.

KAT'S INTERPRETATION

Lou did a great job interpreting his own active diagnostic dream filled with masculine symbolism for prostate cancer. If this were my dream, I would agree that it is a diagnostic dream filled with phallic symbolism. He was draped over the horn, making him vulnerable. Black in a number of the dreams in this book was often a color associated with cancer, as was being chased. Lou had an incredible understanding of a complex dream and used it to save his life.

DR. BURK'S COMMENTARY

Lou has already provided his own insightful interpretation, alluding to the black man as representing an important shadow figure. Although there is no specific mention of the prostate gland or cancer in the dreams, the anatomic location and sense of impending doom are vividly portrayed. Being immersed in water may correlate with a repressed emotion, such as fear in the first chakra. The water element in the Chinese five elements also corresponds to fear and diseases of the bladder and kidneys. While the possibility of rectal or bladder cancer could have been considered, the masculine bull imagery would favor prostate cancer.

Testicular Cancer:
Medical Introduction

Testicular cancer is rare, but still the most common cause of cancer in young men between the ages of 15 and 35. Fortunately, due to early detection, deaths are uncommon. Most cancers are found by discovering a lump through self-examination or examination by a physician. Ultrasound can be used for confirmation, followed by biopsy and treatment by orchiectomy. The blood tests alpha-fetoprotein (AFP) and human chorionic gonadotropin (HCG) can also be used to assist in detecting testicular cancers. In the next story, a warning dream immediately preceded the discovery of the tumor by self-examination.

27

The Playground of Life and Death

Dr. Jay Troutman

I am also a medical doctor and wanted to share my story with you in this book after learning of Dr. Larry Burk's work by watching his TEDx talk on dreams. I am using the pseudonym of Jay Troutman to tell this story.

My Dead Body Dream

I was carrying my dead body and disposing of it in a schoolyard. It felt like the body was made of rubber. As I entered the schoolyard, the kids were playing, which was reminiscent of those days as a child. It forced me to feel like I was on a mission and this body-double needed to go. It was very uncomfortable carrying my body, as it was rubbery and hard to manage. Once I got to the edge of the playground, I threw my body off the side of a ravine.

I woke up shortly after the dream and knew something was very wrong with me. The next day I found my testicular cancer.

Three Unusual Circumstances

The additional story here is that three very unusual circumstances happened that were out of character with my life, and therefore worth mentioning concerning this dream.

The first circumstance was the low-grade depression I had had for the week before detection.

The second happened while performing a skin biopsy on the nose of a young girl. My hands, which are usually very steady, were shaking slightly. Something was happening, and it was unnerving to me. Oddly, after the procedure, which for all intents and purposes should have been traumatic for a young girl, especially on the nose, she looked at me and smiled. Then, with the appearance of a concerned mother, she came over to me and gave me a hug. It was the first time such a thing like this has happened. I remember thinking to myself, as I did with the dream, *Something is wrong with me.*

The third incident involved bathing. I never take baths and had a slight headache, so for whatever reason, I took a bath, the first bath in many months or maybe years. While in the tub, I remembered reading an article about Lance Armstrong, the cyclist who had testicular cancer, and so decided to do the first testicular self-exam I had ever done.

I Found the Tumor

The next day, while at the clinic, I walked over to the urology department and had surgery that night. I thank God every day for the messages that were sent to me. In retrospect, it seems to me that I was throwing away my old life, which is indeed what happened as a result of having cancer. Remarkably, it occurred on the holiday of Lag B'Omer, which in my religion of Judaism is a day of intense spiritual light. I see that day now, and the coincidence of the dream, as a rebirth.

KAT'S INTERPRETATION

If this were my dream I would consider it to be a warning and diagnostic dream showing me what may become of my body in the near future. It is a call-to-action nightmare that was carried over into his waking world. I might think it is happening now because the body looks like the dreamer at the time of the dream, not the body as a child or elderly person.

A *playground* may represent a carefree time in life, devoid of worries or responsibilities and able do as you please. But this playground was in a schoolyard, which is a place of learning. We all carry ourselves through life but seldom look closely at ourselves as we do. Look at the *play on words* the motion picture of the dream presents: "Carry ourselves through the day, or carry on through work." His body was "not feeling right" or looking good to him as he carries it. He then carries himself through his carefree life and discards the life/body into the ravine.

Fortunately, Dr. Troutman understood his dream was a call to action and lived to share it with us.

DR. BURK'S COMMENTARY

Dr. Troutman's dream is ominous but nonspecific in terms of the diagnosis; however, there was other guidance involved beyond the dreamworld that converged in the bathtub upon the Lance Armstrong memory. Many subconscious processes were working in parallel to prompt the simple life-saving act of testicular self-examination, which is well-known to all physicians.

Despite the doctor's training, "Physician heal thyself" is sometimes harder than you might expect, especially at a young age, when you still embrace the illusion of invincibility. Fortunately for men, the examination is more accurate than breast self-examination for women, as reflected in the rarity of deaths from testicular cancer.

Tongue Cancer:
Medical Introduction

Tongue cancer is a form of oral cancer that may present as a sore in the mouth that won't go away or heal completely. The most common type is squamous cell carcinoma, and it may spread to the lymph nodes in the neck. Screening is commonly done during routine dental examinations. Special dyes or lights can assist in detection. These cancers are highly associated with alcohol and tobacco use, but can also be related to human papilloma viral infection.

28

Dead Sucking Insects

Pali Delevitt

Dr. Larry Burk: My friend and former Duke Integrative Medicine colleague Pali Delevitt had lesions on her tongue, but it was dream guidance that eventually led to the diagnosis. She was the most prolific dream journaler I have ever met, and her dreams assisted her in outliving her prognosis by several decades until her eventual death in 2011. Her stories of surviving multiple recurrences due to paying attention to her dreams always enthralled our medical students and prompted my interest in this field of investigation prior to the breast cancer dream project. Here is an excerpt from her book *Wyld Possibilities* about her initial dream diagnosis.[57]

My name is Pali Delevitt and for about a year and a half, painful lesions had been developing on my tongue that were not improving. They had been seen by several doctors who could not clearly diagnose the problem. After a biopsy, and when emerging from my "twilight sleep" under anesthesia, I shared my first conscious thought with the doctor, "You biopsied the wrong part of my tongue." Even as I said it, I thought to myself, "Where did that idea come from?" And, the doctor said, "I am the doctor, and I biopsied the part that needed to be biopsied." When the biopsy came back negative, this was the news that any patient would hope to receive. I was in the clear. However, I began to experience a series of dreams.

Dead Sucking Insects Dream

In the first dream, I found myself regurgitating a pile of dead, sucking insects from my mouth.

Tarantula Spider Dream

A few months later, I dream I am walking into a classroom at the university, sitting down in the professor's chair and preparing to lecture. However, when I opened my mouth, I am unable to speak. Instead, a large tarantula-like black spider crawls out of my lips, down my arm, and sits on my hand, without harming me. I open my mouth once again to speak, and still, no sound comes out. Instead, I had to reach into my mouth and, using my fingers, pull out a mass of sticky white cobwebs left by the spider. When I finally remove it all, I stand up and begin to teach my class.

The lesions did not go away and began to plague me more and more, making it painful to even read aloud to my children at bedtime. I consulted new doctors. When trying to tell them my intuitive sense of what I was experiencing, I got this reply: "My dear, I have been practicing medicine for 27 years, 14 of which was in the Navy. And what medical school did you go to?" Of course, they had already referred to my previous records and the negative biopsy. So once again, I was dismissed with no real diagnosis or treatment.

Hot Lips Houlihan *M.A.S.H.* Dream

Shortly thereafter I had a dream in which I was being examined by the medical staff of the television show *M.A.S.H.* (one of my favorite programs). In the dream, the Harvard-trained Dr. Charles Emerson Winchester and head nurse, Major "Hot Lips" Houlihan, were examining my mouth. They said to me emphatically, "You have a tumor in your tongue that needs to come out immediately!"

One of my doctors finally agreed to do the elective surgery, and when they did, they found a two-millimeter squamous cell cancer embedded in the back of my tongue (not the front, where the doctor had previously biopsied). A few more months and the cancer would have easily metastasized. My dreams were my wakeup call; my inner knowing. They saved my life.

KAT'S INTERPRETATION

Like the dreams Jill Yankee experienced, which appear in the ovarian cancer chapter, Pali's multiple dreams also use the symbol of the *spider*, very similar to a crab, as a sign for cancer. If this were my dream, I would define it as an active, recurrent, symbolic diagnostic dream. Although the exact dream itself is not recurrent, the message is repetitive and is offered differently multiple times. A *white-coated doctor* may mean the dream deals with a medical issue. *Losing her voice* in the dream and finding it difficult to speak in her waking life may have been a duality, indicative of the loss of her power to the doctors, which may be reflective of the fifth chakra, which is the voice chakra.

Pali's dreams spoke to her in her own dream language of *Hot Lips Houlihan*, a very strong female living in a man's *M.A.S.H.* world and Dr. Winchester, one of the show's best yet more challenging doctors with whom to work.

DR. BURK'S COMMENTARY

Pali's dreams featured insects and spiders as symbols of cancer in a fashion similar to many others, with the mouth being the actual location in her case. The persistent messages, including ones from fictional dream medical professionals, made her persist in pursuing the diagnosis, despite resistance from her doctors. White-coated physicians were one of the most common dream messengers in the Breast Cancer Dreams Project. It is great to have access to this type of second opinion. It is also important when initial biopsies or imaging studies are negative to continue to follow the dream guidance.

Uterine Cancer:
Medical Introduction

U terine cancer is the fourth most common cancer in women, and it is rising in incidence due to the increase in obesity, a risk factor for the disease. Other risk factors include menses before age 12, menopause after age 55, estrogen therapy, and family history. Since it begins inside the uterus, it does not show up on a Pap test, so other signs like abnormal bleeding are important warnings.

29

Giving Birth

Ann Charles

Dr. Larry Burk: My close friend Ann Charles is a retired MRI
technologist who has had many guiding dreams during her life. She
is also a biofeedback therapist, a hypnotherapist, an energy healer,
and a skilled rug hooker. When she heard about my cancer dream
research and upcoming TEDx talk in 2016, she told me about her
recent experience with the dream diagnosis of uterine cancer.

Giving Birth Dream

I had a dream about giving birth, which made no sense because I am post-
menopausal, so it was impossible.

My thought was perhaps it might be a metaphor for giving birth to a creative project, since I am an artist always coming up with new inspirations,
sometimes in dreams. However, it might be a warning of a physical illness in my
uterus, although I had no symptoms.

A Question Answered by a Clarifying Dream

As an experienced dreamer, I knew what to do next and asked for a clarifying
dream the following night.

The Graveyard Dream

I got what I asked for, which was a very disturbing dream of being taken to
a graveyard in Ireland to a see a headstone surrounded by daisies. I heard a
dream voice say that if I didn't act on the guidance from the previous dream,
I would be pushing up those daisies soon.

My gynecologist ordered an ultrasound that showed an endometrial carcinoma. Shortly afterward, a vaginal hysterectomy was performed, where the
tumor was removed surgically through my vagina, symbolically mirroring the
delivery process in the first dream. I made a complete recovery and am cancer-
free, thanks to my dream guidance.

KAT'S INTERPRETATION

Ann's story elicited an ASMR (Autonomous Sensory Meridian Response) from me, as discussed in the Preface. I concur with Dr. Larry Burk that the more bizarre the dream, the stronger the message, and asking for clarification is often the best way to get a clear answer. If this were my dream, I would define it as both a literal and symbolic diagnostic dream. What is so interesting about her dreams is that they were giving the dreamer much the same message in two different ways. The first dream was symbolic. When Ann did not get it, the second dream was literal, with a voiced warning of "pushing up daisies." It is amazing how many dreams nagged the dreamers until the message was understood. I might also see the dream of giving birth as birthing a new and healthy life.

DR. BURK'S COMMENTARY

Ann's story again reminds us of the dilemma of differentiating a metaphorical dream from a dream of a real physical illness, as in the case of Aisha Umar. The first dream indicated a physical location indirectly through the act of giving birth, but made no indication of cancer or severe disease. Fortunately, the request for the clarifying dream was fulfilled in dramatic fashion. It is a cautionary tale about not ignoring dream guidance just because it comes in a puzzling form. In fact, often the dreams that seem most bizarre contain the most relevant information, presented in an unusual way to get our attention. Remembering to ask for a clarifying dream the next night, when you are perplexed with one in the morning, is a useful talent to cultivate.

PART FOUR

Developing Your Own Dream Skills

30

Ways to Remember Your Dreams

Kathleen (Kat) O'Keefe-Kanavos

A dream which is not interpreted
is like a letter which is not read.
— The Talmud

Have you met your Physician-within yet? Set the intention to meet this important part of your life tonight before going to sleep. My Physician-within introduced herself during a dream as Dr. Jules (or Jewels, as a play on words, because she is a real jewel), and the information she imparted about my three cancers five years before they were discovered and shown as three crabs saved my life as discussed in Part II: Chapter 14.

Finding cancer in dreams missed three times by the medical field and the tests on which they rely is as lucky as winning the lottery three times in a row. Luck had little to do with it; it was divine intervention.

Mistakes happen. Science only goes so far, then comes your Higher Power, often in dreams. However, the dream with my Physician-within, Dr. Jules, and the three crabs did not come to full fruition for five years. By journaling my dreams, I was able to go back and research my dreams for additional validation and outcome.

As an R.A. Boch Cancer Hotline phone counselor, I've found that my story is unusual but not unique. Many women told me that they had had dreams about their cancer but did not take them seriously. What makes my story special is that I believed and followed my dreams. There is almost always a point in the process of illness where logic, reason, and medical expertise fail. It is at this point that a patient can slip through the cracks, often never to recover.[58] We hold all of the answers to our well-being within; dreams are the keys to the solution.

Dreams have been around since cave dwellers drew on the walls. The Talmud (AD 56) says that a dream not remembered is like a letter unread. Think of your dreams as love letters from Inner Guidance. We may not realize how much we love ourselves until a dream saves our life.

Do you ever wake up exhausted after a long night's sleep and wonder why you feel like you just ran a marathon? You may be doing dreamwork that contains guidance and answers to daily concerns or desires. Our dreams are a "safe zone," where we can work out solutions to daily challenges and not be judged or arrested for uncivilized behavior.[59] We can misbehave in a dream to blow off steam from a stressful workplace, and it is okay. We won't get fired or arrested and thrown in jail, or if we do in the dream, we get out when we wake up.

When you awaken ask yourself, *What did I learn?* Remembering your dream is paramount to learning, implementing, and benefiting from the dream information.[60]

One of the biggest challenges many of us face concerning dreamwork is retaining our dream information. It does not matter how many dream dictionaries we have or how many dream journals we keep if our dreams are too elusive to remember. We must learn to remember not to forget. Holding onto dreams after turning off the alarm clock is a learned skill.

Imagine your mind flexing like fingers as they are gently caressing your butterfly-like dreams before they can fly away. Build your mind-muscle with dream exercises provided in this chapter. Remember: use it or lose it.

This chapter shares easy, tried-and-true dream memory methods, which I used while undergoing surgery, chemotherapy, and radiation treatment for breast cancer and which will help you receive and retrieve life-saving information. If you have a challenge or concern, "sleep on it" to find the solution.

SO DREAM

I used the seven-letter acronym SO DREAM to remind me of the seven steps needed to retrieve my dreams and information.

These are as follows:

S=SET YOUR INTENTION, which is a dream part of the Law of Attraction. An intention is the first step in attracting and manifesting information. A simple request is all it takes. *I wish to meet my Physician-within or get a solution to* (fill in the blank) *in my dream tonight.* Or, it can be something as simple as, *I want to remember my dream.*

Write your intention on a piece of paper and place it under your pillow to "sleep on it," a play on words that holds profound meaning. By doing this, you are also showing your inner self, through your eyes (considered the windows to the soul), what you intend to do: take a dream from the abstract fifth dimension and bring it into the concrete third dimension of life by turning it into written words that contain messages.

O=**ORGANIZE** yourself before sleep to record your dream upon awakening. Put your dream journal, pen, or recording device (and a flashlight, if necessary) by your bed. If your dream awakens you, it may be telling you to write down or record relevant information before you forget it. This often happens with multiple dreams. If you get up to hunt for a pencil or paper, you may lose your dream.

D= **DREAM**, in order to begin the process of fulfilling your intention. Studies have shown that all living things dream, including you, because you began to dream in the womb at seven months.[61] Dreaming is the first step in training your brain to remember dreams.

R=**REMAIN** in your same sleep position when you first awaken to **remember** and **record** whatever you can of your dream. Moving around may cause your dream to dissolve like the morning shadows. Use this step to reenter your dream state at a later time to retrieve additional information. More information on this topic is provided in the next chapter.

E=**EMOTION** refers to those parts of the dream, or snippets, that **elicit** emotion—that stick in your mind and create a physical response, such as rapid breathing, cold sweats, tears, or a pounding heart.

A=**ADD** to your dream memory by asking, *What colors, sounds, words, people, animals, plants, signs, and symbols did I see? What names and phrases did I hear?* They may be an important part of the meaning in your message that fulfills your intention. If more of the dream returns during the day, jot it down on a piece of paper or record it on your phone to add to your journal later. This can help you with dream tracking: keeping track of dreams, messages, and images to see if they come true.

M=**MEANING**. What do the small dream parts known as snippets mean to you? Dreams are as individual as the dreamer. What is important to you in a dream may be unimportant to someone else because it does not elicit the same emotion. Pictures, forms, creatures, colors, lack of colors, people, and phrases are all part of your individual dream language. It is one of many ways we communicate with ourselves.

Put the information from the acronym SO DREAM together, start dream tracking, and begin developing your dream language. If the dream is still confusing, ask for a clarifying dream the following night, as some of the dreamers in the book did.

Finally, give your dream a title, even if it's *The Dream Without a Name*, so if part of it returns during the day, you will know where to add it in your journal.

Our dreams often use a play on words to speak to us. "Washing your hands" of a situation, "kicking something around" in the dream are examples that come to mind of working out a solution or ridding yourself of a problem as a means of solving a challenge.

So, tonight, dream on your intention, and remember not to forget your dream.

Your dreams are an incredible tool to help you overcome or work through any illness or crisis with guided healing information for a healthier and more fulfilled life. The trick is remembering them, so you can distinguish them from other dream types that may convey a message. If necessary, you can reenter a dream in order to get further information, as described in the next chapter.

31

Reentering Your Dreams to Retrieve Information

Kathleen (Kat) O'Keefe-Kanavos

"Life is tricky. Embrace your magic."

Have you ever awakened and thought, *I didn't finish my dream and want to get back into it.* Or, *What was the information I needed to remember from my dream?* It may be a perfect opportunity to reenter your dream. Creating or changing the ending of your dream may be therapeutic and shift your life.

The names associated with the following dream have been modified to respect the privacy request of the dreamer calling into my radio show, although the dream was told to me and recorded during my live show, with the full knowledge of the dreamer, who then became a client.

Linda was distraught because she kept having a recurring nightmare that woke her in the middle of the night. It was serious because it was affecting all aspects of her life, including her health.

Knock. Knock. Who's There? Dream

Linda was dreaming when there would be a knock on a door. (The knock was her signal that the dream had shifted and was lucid and recurrent.) She realized that she was again sitting on the couch in her living room, watching TV with her husband. As the knock from across the room persisted, her husband stood to answer it.

Linda would yell, "No! Don't open the door!"

But her husband would walk across the dark living room and open it, anyway.

Standing on the other side of the threshold was her deceased father, who would walk into the room and say, "Linda, I love you."

Linda's father's words would jolt her from the dream and leave her upset for the rest of the day because she and her father had had a terrible relationship while he was alive.

"He was mean and made my life miserable. He never told me he loved me while he was alive. Not once! Why does he keep coming into my dreams now to tell me he loves me? I can't stand him, can't take this anymore, and I'm afraid to go to sleep. I lost my job because I missed work so much from exhaustion, I don't feel well, and my marriage is on the rocks because I am always in a bad mood. What can I do to make my dad leave me alone? Why is he showing up now after all these years? I hate him!"

"Well, Linda," I said, "perhaps the little girl in you still loves Daddy, or you would not be this upset by his words, 'I love you.' How badly do you want the dreams to stop?"

"I'll do anything!" she said.

"Okay. Set the intention before you go to sleep each night that if you have this nightmare, you will not wake up until you have changed the ending and resolved the issue. The next time you have the dream, hold yourself in it. If you exit the dream, stay in the same sleeping position, breathe, and slide back into the dream. When you hear the knock on the door, *you* get up and answer it. And when your dad says, 'Linda, I love you.' You tell him you love him, too."

"But I don't love him. I can't stand him. I can't do that!"

"How badly do you want these nightmares to stop?"

After a long pause, Linda said, "Okay."

Two weeks passed, and I did not hear from Linda. Her silence was worrisome. Did she not have the recurrent nightmare yet, or did she have it and explode from anger?

Almost on cue, the phone rang. It was Linda talking a mile a minute.

"You'll never believe what happened the night after we spoke. I set my intention before I went to sleep."

In my dream, I heard the knock on the door and almost ran out of my dream, but told myself to stay, and I did. When my husband got up, I told him to let me answer the door. I had to really focus on not waking up as I crossed the dark living room to open the door.

My dad was standing there. He looked at me and said, "Linda, I love you."

Kat, I don't know what came over me, but I threw my arms around his neck and said, "Daddy, I love you, too."

And while I was holding him he disappeared.

"I have not seen or heard from him since. That was two weeks ago. That is the longest I have not had this dream. What happened?"

"Well, first of all, you just verbally shifted your nightmare into a healing dream for you and your father. You reentered your dream to change the ending, and it has already changed your life. No one in the world can challenge us like our parents, either dead or alive. If the problems don't kill us, they make us stronger. When our family dies, they are given opportunities to see how they affected the lives of their loved ones. That is their learning experience on the other side.

"The Rule of Permission is powerful and highly respected on the other side. Your dad could not return to atone for his mistreatment of you without the authorization from his Higher Power. He knocked on the door (asking permission). Your husband, whom I have heard you refer to as your "better half," answered the door for you. But facing your father (play on words) was something *you* had to do.

"When you opened your door to your home, you rekindled a heart connection with your father. Sometimes, actions speak louder than words and love is all you need, because love is something you can take with you. Love transcends time, space, and death. The therapeutic intention of reentering your dream and changing your ending allowed you to solve the problem."

Linda said she felt wonderful when she woke up. A simple hug of love changed the ending of a lucid nightmare into a healing dream that transformed her life forever.

KAT'S INTERPRETATION

If this were my dream, I would call it a lucid, symbolic, and literal healing dream. In dreams, a *home* is your body, and the *living room* is where you live. It is a play on words. A *knock on a door* is asking permission, often between realms. The words *I love you* are incredibly powerful, because they can heal a broken heart. Linda carried the anger of not being told she was loved all her life until the fateful knock on the door, which was also a wakeup call: "Yes, you are loved, and it is better you know that later than never." But, most importantly, Linda learned to reenter her lucid dream to manifest a different positive ending.

We dream for many reasons. Here are three important ones.
1. Entertainment and relaxation
2. Problem solving
3. Receiving answers to a question set by an intention

Benefits to Reentering Your Dreams

How well do you know your inner guides or spirit guides in dreams? Tallulah Lyons and I are in constant contact with both. We combined our personal experiences and shared them as one of 24 presentations at the International Association for the Study of Dreams (IASD) 2014 PsiberDreaming Conference Symposium, *Dreaming with the Other.*

The goal of this online symposium was to explore and share cutting-edge research and information on dreams, spirit guides, and dreaming with the other. The information was then shared with medical practitioners, students, mystics, metaphysicians, and the world community of dreamers. We helped dream group members integrate their healing dream imagery.

One of the ways this is most effective for anyone overcoming cancer treatment is through integrative practices that include dream therapy or dream groups offered in cancer centers. Guided imagery, mindfulness meditation, yoga, tai chi, expressive art, and music are all grounded in a meditative state of consciousness. Using the meditative practice of dream reentry through self-guided imagery can be beneficial to a dreamer seeking guidance.

Nightmares can be a blessing in disguise and a call to action. Dreams that frighten us and awaken us in the middle of the night usually contain an important message. Disturbing our sleep is a way of telling us not to forget what is important in our dream world for our waking life. Unfortunately, an abrupt awakening can cause us to feel confused and forget the dream.

Dreamers are encouraged to enter or reenter a dream or nightmare with the intention to:

1. Allow their relationship to continue, so the issues in the dream can transform.
2. Allow dreamers to side-step rational thought and verbal interpretation.
3. Take the dreamer into a safe space between consciousness and unconsciousness.
4. Immerse the dreamer in a journey of emotional sensations and facilitate a direct encounter with elements of the dream that need transformation.

Meditation is also a form of lucid daydreaming. This approach allows for a shift at an embodied level as well as transformation of mind and spirit.

Steps to Reenter Your Dreams

Why would you ever want to reenter a bad dream or nightmare? Don't we prefer to forget the unpleasant? One of the important reasons to reenter a dream is to allow the relationships in your dream to grow and develop in a positive manner. Our nightmares can be a blessing in disguise and a call to action, as seen in Linda's nightmare. This was also addressed previously in Benefits to Reentering Your Dream.

Here are steps practiced by Tallulah and me on how to reenter your dream for clarification, contact, and retrieval of forgotten information.

If awakening unexpectedly from a dream, resettle into the same sleep position and then:

1. Follow the breath into a deeply relaxed state.
2. Enter an imaginal healing sanctuary.
3. Invite your inner guide.
4. Reenter the dream from a new perspective of remaining grounded in support and guidance and let the elements of the dream move and shift at will.
5. Allow new insights, perspectives, and interactions to unfold.
6. Imagine any transformed imagery as healing energy.
7. Imagine sending the healing energy into any part of the body, mind, or spirit in need of special tuning.

Dream journaling is an excellent source for researching personal dream dilemma and information. Dream tracking keeps track of dreams that may be recurrent or important. You can highlight questions or dream events and reenter dreams to research the answers.

Not all dreams are filled with life-altering information that must be remembered. However, when you are in crisis or plan to make the mistake of a lifetime, what I call our "ET (Eternal Teacher) phones home" for help. Dreams are phone lines to the other side.

Spirit guides send information, often heard as words, through dreams that not only diagnose illness but can diagnose and guide you toward a creative relationship with all aspect of your life.

Reentering dreams is an excellent way to dialogue with self and your spirit guides.

PART FIVE

*True Dreams of Other
Non-Cancer Illnesses*

Dreams may contain ineluctable truths, philosophical pronouncements,
illusions, wild fantasies, memories, plans, anticipations, irrational
experiences, even telepathic visions, and heaven knows what besides.
— CARL JUNG, *CW 8, Para 317*

Welcome to the personal stories of dreams that impacted the lives of other people who were not part of Dr. Larry Burk's Breast Cancer Dream Project but shared many of the same life-saving results from their precognitive, healing, diagnostic, and lucid dreams. The following stories of dreams of ordinary people are extraordinary examples of how we are all connected to Universal Oneness and the Sacred Dream Doorways to Universal Guidance.

32

Bike Injury Warning Dream

Larry Burk, MD, CEHP

The week after my 60th birthday, in early December 2015, I had a disturbing early morning dream.

> I was driving a car in unsafe conditions, when the woman in the passenger seat said someone had predicted she would have an NDE today. Heeding her warning, I drove extra carefully through a construction zone, but in the next scene I wound up in a hospital bed thinking that I had had a stroke because my whole left side was damaged. The neurologist came in and asked if I had any actual neurological symptoms. I moved my arm and leg and said no, and he said I would be fine and could go home right away.

I woke up and found the dream concerning, but attempted to avoid dealing with it by not telling my wife Dagmar, which is unusual for me as we often share dreams in the morning.

We went out for a morning bike ride before breakfast in 39-degree weather to test our brand new thermal winter biking gear with three laps of our road. I decided to ride very cautiously due to the dream warning and the cold conditions, in case there was any black ice left over from the frigid night. However, we didn't have winter gloves, only our summer ones with the fingertips cut out, so my fingers got very cold. After two laps of careful riding, I had the ingenious idea of putting my right hand in my pocket to stay warm.

Going down the first hill on the third lap, I realized I was going too fast and squeezed the left handle for the front brake without squeezing the right handle for the back brake, something every experienced biker knows not to do. The front tire locked abruptly. I flew over the left handlebar and hit the asphalt on a stretch of the road that was undergoing repair.

I landed on my left shoulder, left elbow, and left hip and bounced right back up without broken bones, only some severe bruises. I remembered that the dream neurologist said I would be fine, so I got back on the bike and finished the last lap home. After taking multiple doses of the homeopathic remedy Arnica Montana, I healed up relatively uneventfully in a week or two.

KAT'S INTERPRETATION

If this were my dream I would give it to Larry to analyze because he did such a great job of uncovering all the little golden nuggets of information hidden in the dream. It was precognitive because it showed a problem or event in the future. The *car* might be seen as his body, the *woman* in the car may have been his inner female balance or his wife. The *construction site* in the dream may have been the place to watch for in the waking world as the site of the upcoming accident. Larry's *Physician-within* may have been the neurologist with a message, telling Larry he was fine and to go home.

DR. BURK'S COMMENTARY

I was amazed at how accurately the dream four hours before had predicted my being injured on my left side and escaping serious damage, but was puzzled by the meaning of the dream. As a warning dream it was ineffective, as it almost seemed like a self-fulfilling prophecy despite my efforts at riding safely. Upon further reflection, it occurred to me that by putting my right hand in my pocket, which is connected to my left brain I took my rational thinking offline. Then my left hand, which is connected to my right brain, created the accident—not what I would expect my intuitive wisdom to do, as it usually has a protective function.

Wondering what the lesson was in the experience, I realized it was about resilience. I had just turned 60 and was able to survive a bad bike accident with only a few bruises, instead of winding up in the operating room with a broken hip or worse. As it turned out, it was a timely message.

Several months later, in March 2016, I was overwhelmed from dealing with breast cancer recurrences with my mother and sister when my application to do a TEDx talk on "Cancer Warning Dreams that Can Save Your Life" was accepted, which entailed several weeks of intense preparation. Fortunately, I was feeling resilient enough to get through that month successfully and give the talk which, ironically, was later censored by TED for being too far outside their traditional scientific guidelines. You can still watch the video at *www.larryburkmd.com* under the Integrative Medicine links by clicking on the X in the upper right corner of the red banner to remove it.

33

Whose Broken Bones?

Patricia Rose Upczak

Throughout my life, I have had vivid, colorful dreams. As a child, I assumed everybody's experience was the same as mine.

When I was in the second grade, a nun overheard me telling a friend about a colorful dream I had had the night before. She reprimanded me for lying. She said in front of the whole class, "People don't dream in color."

To this day, I can remember how confused and angry I was. "Well, I do!" I said determinedly. "And I am not lying. I have always dreamed in color."

So the nun wanted to show the class I was wrong and asked them to raise their hand if they ever dreamed in color. Much to her surprise and my relief, a number of students raised their hands.

Along with dreaming in color, I have had a number of what are called pre-cognitive dreams—dreams that show the future and come true. Some of these were easy to understand, some were symbolic, and some I didn't comprehend until the event happened later.

Over 20 years ago I had a vivid dream just before I woke up one fall morning. This dream tried to protect me from a great deal of pain and discomfort.

The first image was a large royal blue X-ray of a woman's shoulder. The next image was of my good friend Dorothe in the background of the dream.
So when I woke up, I decided I needed to call Dorothe later that day and warn her about a possible fall or something connected to her shoulder.

I called Dorothe, told her about my dream, and that she was in it. My brilliant deduction was Dorothe or one of her grown daughters or a close friend might break their shoulder. I warned her and went on about my very hectic life.

Six weeks later, I tripped over my large black Labrador Retriever and hit my shoulder on a sharp wooden corner near the staircase.

The next morning, my pain was so excruciating I went to the doctor. The dream still eluded me until the doctor brought out the X-ray. The picture was exactly like the arm break in my dream. I had broken the ball of the humerus bone. For years, I could not understand why I had had a dream I didn't comprehend and that didn't help me avoid breaking my shoulder.

Well, recently all the clues came together, and it really surprised me because of all the parts that completely escaped me.

My friend Dorothe was a world-famous clairvoyant before she died a few years ago. When I first met her in 1984, she had told me the essence of my soul was royal blue. She never really told me what it meant, nor did we ever really talk about it much afterward. It was just part of my original reading from her way back then. Well, just recently I found the paper with my notes from the reading and stared at the line about the royal blue essence of my spirit. Clues started to complete the riddle of the dream.

The X-ray in my dream was a vivid royal blue, and I knew it was a woman who was going to get hurt. Dorothe in the background of the dream was symbolic. Seeing her was supposed to guide me to the conclusion the X-ray belonged to me because of its color clue. The clue I missed completely was that Dorothe had told me about my royal blue vibration. The royal blue X-ray was the connection that really had not occurred to me.

Over the years I have had a number of dreams filled with symbols that were able to be worked out and understood. I have collaborated with the incredible Denise Linn around dreams and thought I was very good at figuring out what the symbols meant. So this dream actually has always fascinated and frustrated me because I just didn't understand why I had had it if it wasn't going to tell me clearly that the shoulder belonged to me. Apparently, the dream had sent the right message; I just didn't get it until now. Well, better late than never.

KAT'S INTERPRETATION

If this were my dream, I would define it as a warning precognitive dream that came true because it showed a future condition. Patricia saw an X-ray of a broken bone in the dream and after breaking her bone saw the same X-ray. This dream uses symbolism, which caused confusion in the dreamer's interpretation.

The *color blue* was the color of Patricia's vibration, but it is also the color of the sixth chakra, also known as the third eye/inner-intuition chakra. Perhaps her intuition was also speaking to her, making this dream a duality concerning the color blue.

DR. BURK'S COMMENTARY

This dream highlights the challenge of determining whether a dream is warning you about a personal issue or whether you are dreaming about someone else. Asking for a clarifying dream, as Ann did in Chapter 29, may be useful in this situation of uncertainty. Also, when a precognitive dream of trauma comes true, despite a compelling warning, it raises the question of whether the future can actually be changed by taking a different course of action. If not, then perhaps the dreamer will at least be better prepared to deal with the consequences of the trauma, albeit with a sense of frustration about not being able to prevent it.

34

Deadly Sweet Dreams of Type 2 Diabetes

Maria Mars

In 2014, I was diagnosed with type 2 diabetes. During the year leading up to the diagnosis, I had a series of dreams which, interpreted literally, point to the imbalanced process taking place in my body with respect to blood sugar management. At the same time, the illness was making itself known, and I was experiencing significant change and loss in almost all aspects of my life—career, relationships, finances, identity, and so on. Looking back at these dreams, in particular, it is now apparent they were calling for awareness not only of the emotional-spiritual aspects of my life but the physical as well.

Before diagnosis, I had begun to experience digestive issues (which may or may not be related to diabetes). The problems continued to increase once treated with medication. Though not provided below, there have been countless dreams on the theme of dysfunctional toilets.

January 24, 2013: Dream Doctor

A white male doctor of modern medicine approaches me to discuss certain patient conditions and diagnoses. He is seeking information about diseases and their symbolic relationships.

NOTES: This appears to be the first dream indicating the possible presence of a physical illness with a spiritual/emotional relationship. The dream thread continues throughout the night, as I repeatedly awaken from conversations with the dream doctor. The next two dreams are among a total of five dreams remembered and recorded that night. Two of them appear related to the emerging physical condition.

Blood Dream

I am at the workplace and manipulating an image projected onto a screen. The image is a red fluid. It is blood that has been watered down so that it moves effortlessly and without resistance.

NOTES: This dream seems to point to healing a condition often experienced by people who have Type 2 diabetes and who may or may not have been diagnosed: hyperglycemic hyperosmolar syndrome. It is often described as "thick blood," caused by a severely elevated blood sugar concentration. The dream indicates that this condition may be manageable or controllable, as the blood is "watered down."

Boston Creams Dreams

I am in the staff lounge at work. Someone has provided a box of Boston cream doughnuts. A colleague decides she will take them all home and puts them into a sealable plastic bag. I think it's unfair for her to enjoy them all, so I take the bag and hide it.

NOTES: This dream is pointing to both diabetes and the desire to benefit from the sweetness of life, but the inability to do so at that time – hiding the sweetness. I am envious of others who are able to embrace joy/sweetness and feel deserving of it.

February 10, 2013: Party Platter Dream

I am standing in a large hall with many long tables placed within it. A party is happening, with many people milling about. Place settings are waiting on the tables, as well as baskets stuffed with all sorts of desserts—pastries, cookies, cakes, candies. I pick up a grand food platter, place every single dessert on it, and walk around serving and offering sweets to the partygoers. They can select from "everything." The second time I make my way around the room, the dessert supply is less abundant, with a smaller quantity and less selection of desserts. I feel panicked. While people are away from the tables, I walk up a few steps to the stage and into a dark room behind a door.

NOTES: It seems I am at the party yet unable to enjoy it with the others. I take up the role of serving sweets (joy, happiness) to others in the room. I am not eating the sugary treats myself, yet when I am unable to provide more sweetness to the others, I retreat and hide. Again, there is a parallel between the physical condition and the spiritual/emotional. At that time in my life, I was not providing sweetness/joy for my own life but instead allowing others to define happiness for me. When I could no longer be sweet in their midst, I withdrew from the relationships.

February 18, 2013: Syrupy Sweet Apples Dream

Some girlfriends come over for a visit and a chat. I look for munchies in the kitchen cupboard and find a stash of flavored rice crackers. I put them into a bowl, and they turn into candy. I then find tiny green apples in the cupboard, and I am about to put them out when I notice they are now covered in a thick red syrup. One of my friends takes a bite from a syrupy apple and raves about its sweetness. I try to rinse the syrup off the apples, but the apple skins adopt the reddish hue of the syrup, and they still taste so much sweeter than their sour or tart flavor. I am unable to restore them to their essential state.

NOTES: Foods turning directly into refined sugars. They are too sweet for me, and my sense of taste rejects them, though my girlfriends are able to eat and enjoy the sugar.

Dream Snippets

I experience numerous dream fragments between this time and August 30, 2014. They all seem to reflect choices between this food and that food, such as milk instead of flour, strawberries instead of wheat, green bananas instead of overripe bananas, a semi-sweet dessert bun instead of an all-out sugar fest, and so on.

August 30, 2014: Corn Skeletons Dream

I am standing at the edge of a cornfield, looking at rows upon rows of golden corn stalks. As I stand there, the stalks begin to dry out. Then the stalks turn into blackened skeletons.

NOTES: The initial association to corn was HFCS (high-fructose corn syrup), one of the sweeteners added to and hidden in many processed foods. There may be a link between HFCS and diabetes. This dream seemed to be a warning to stay away from corn products, and HFCS in particular. Much later, a year and a half later, I noticed another association to the rapid drying of the corn stalks in the dream and the chemical "glyphosate," an ingredient in the herbicide Roundup. Farmers are encouraged to use this as a desiccant or drying agent in order to generate a higher yield and increase profit. Glyphosate has been implicated in gut flora imbalances, inflammation, irritable bowel syndrome, and so on, which were formerly attributed to gluten intolerance.

At the time that these dreams were recorded, I was not interpreting them from a literal perspective, asking myself, "Could this happen in real life?" as I learned to do later in an active dreaming course with Robert Moss. It was only after the diagnosis and review of my dreams that it became quite clear what the dream messengers were trying to alert me to from a multidimensional perspective.

KAT'S INTERPRETATION

If these were my dreams, I would define them as a combination of guided and diagnostic, which were also active, literal, and symbolic. The male doctor acted as a Physician-within while he conversed with Maria and asked questions, which made the interaction literal and active. Her dreams are also symbolic, as seen with the *red blood*, which may be interpreted as raw, powerful life force. Red is a powerful color and blood is a life force. Watching your life on a screen may be seen as viewing yourself from the inside out. I would add to Maria's ideas that the party platter dream, where she served desserts to her inner selves, was not going to happen, and it upset her because one of the fun things in life is a sweet party. Maria has a strong understanding of how she is being guided to understand a health crisis conclusion.

DR. BURK'S COMMENTARY

It is intriguing that her first dream mentions a white male doctor interested in the symbolic meaning of diseases, as that is an accurate description of me and my passion for exploring metaphorical illnesses and healing in my coaching practice and writings. I wonder if it may have been precognitive of her contributing this chapter for the book. I teach my coaching clients who are dealing with diabetes to question why they don't make their life sweeter instead of their blood. Her dreams seem to be providing this lesson for her.

Diabetes can also be considered a severe imbalance of the earth element in the Traditional Chinese Medicine theory of the five elements, impacting the energy flow to the spleen and pancreas. The challenge of the earth element is to know how to nurture oneself while also nurturing others, as she highlights in one of her dreams. Sugar is considered damaging to the spleen in Chinese medicine, but unfortunately, sweet confections are a common way of expressing affection and celebration in our culture. It is a tradition that is exploited by the food industry around every holiday, so it is little wonder that sugar is considered a substitute for happiness, despite its detrimental effect on our health.

Warning! Do Not Have Sex

Athena Kolinski

It has always been my practice to get tested between sexual partners, to protect myself and others. Well, this was the first time in a long time I had not
followed my own protocol.

When I met "the new guy," things happened so fast I didn't get to that part—
you know, get tested or protect myself. As with all new sexual relationships,
things got hot and heavy with the excitement and newness. About two weeks
after meeting him, I had this dream.

Warning: Do Not Have Sex!

I dreamt of my last long-term lover, whom I had stopped seeing about six
months earlier. I wanted to have sex with him again but then I remembered
I was involved with a new guy. At some point, someone told me, "You have
something. Whatever you do, do not have sex with a new partner until you
get tested."

I woke up from the dream freaked out. I'm not sure how much more literal the
message could be. However, I had absolutely no signs or symptoms of anything
being medically wrong.

The next few days I spent calming myself down and had a conversation
with my new lover about our terms and conditions. We had agreed from the
forefront that there would be other people in our lives, but I asked him a few
more specific questions about his safety habits. Everything seemed up to par,
so I let go of the concern.

Two weeks after the dream, I ended up with a rash you know where that
was like nothing I had ever experienced in my life.

Intuitively, I began to put the pieces together. I had left a tampon in overnight for 10 hours, something I never do. I had both slept with the tampon in
and kept it in for a long duration. For several days, an image in my head kept
appearing of the terrible rash that developed after my knee surgery a few years

earlier from being exposed to glue for several days. Since the surgery, I had grown hypersensitive to Band-Aids, kinesthetic tape, stickers, and basically anything with glue on it. Within an hour of glue touching my skin, I would be red, irritated, and uncomfortable.

At the medical office, the doctor went straight to the worst-case scenario to prepare me for the test results. I couldn't believe that he wouldn't even consider that this was an allergic reaction to the glue in the tampon and pads. Five days later my rash was not getting better, so I went to urgent care for a second opinion, knowing they would give me faster test results.

There, every test under the sun run was run on me. Three days later, all the results came back negative for every possible STD (sexually transmitted disease) scenario. It was exactly as my intuition had told me: I am allergic to the glue in the feminine products.

Although I did not have any issues when I had the dream, it did clue me in to the fact I needed to not add anyone else into the mix. Prior to the scare, it also led me to have a deeper conversation with my new lover to ensure we were on the same sexual page, which gave me more peace of mind when the rash appeared.

Of course, when it did appear, my mind went straight back to the dream, making me think I must have contracted something during the intimate part of my new relationship. But that thought was what most people's minds, including the doctor's, would immediately jump to. However, I didn't have an STD; I had an allergic reaction. I am so thankful that I trusted my own instincts around the situation and did not take the medication that was prescribed or accept the doctor's worst-case scenario as truth.

There were thoughts of what my life would look like if it were the worst-case scenario, but I didn't let that thought overtake me.

Mostly the dream and the incident taught me that I needed to go back to asking the tough questions around intimacy safety and STD testing right up front, ensuring safety and respect for all parties involved. And to trust my dreams.

KAT'S INTERPRETATION

If this were my dream, I would define it as a warning dream that was literal. It was not about symbolism; it was about listening to the dream's advice.

DR. BURK'S COMMENTARY

This story is an excellent example of the intersection between intuition and dream guidance in navigating through a delicate relationship issue. If in our culture, families restored the time-honored tradition of dream sharing at breakfast, perhaps more of our younger generations would be better prepared for accessing their inner wisdom to inform such important decisions.

36

"I Sprang a Leak" and "I Blew a Fuse"

Kathi Kemper, MD, MPH

My name is Dr. Kathi Kemper, and I have two dreams that came true to share with you.

The first dream I had was as a medical student.

"I Sprang a Leak"

In the dream, my car's radiator had overheated and sprung a leak.

The next day, there was no problem with my car; however, I did develop a fever and a urinary tract infection that made me feel as if I had "sprung a leak." This has made me pay more attention to the subtle cues of my own dreams.

Recently a friend let me try a pulsed electromagnetic field device, an expensive one, for a few days to see if it would help with some symptoms I had. I followed the directions exactly and didn't really feel anything. On the third day, I had a dream.

"I Blew a Fuse"

I was in my "dream house" and walking upstairs; I ran into the electrician who was working on the circuits in an upper-floor room. He sternly warned me NOT to turn on the electricity again until he had finished his repairs or I'd risk blowing out the whole house and starting a fire.

Based on this dream, I stopped using the device immediately and returned it to my friend. It may be helpful for others but was not right for me. A few days later, my heart rate variability (a measure of overall well-being), which had dropped a bit during the days I'd used the device, rebounded to normal, confirming the wisdom of the dream.

KAT'S INTERPRETATION

When I read Dr. Kathi Kemper's dream about the electromagnetic field device to Lori Boyle, my iPhone, lying on the table pretty far away, without being touched or prompted, turned itself on and contacted "Siri," the smartphone's electronic assistant app, which read the dream back to me. It freaked us both out, but gave me the chance to write the dream down, word for word. Thanks, Siri.

If these were my dreams, I would call the first one a symbolic healing dream, as our *car* often symbolizes our body and may show a larger, future health issue if the dream were not taken seriously.

I would describe the second dream as a literal and symbolic guided diagnostic dream, with the *wires in your house* being the veins and electrical current in your body, and the *electrician* as an *inner-diagnostician*, trying to fix the inner wiring of the body. The dream was literal, because the electrician spoke and gave specific guided directions (Definitely don't use the electromagnetic field device again). But the best part of the dream to me was the electrician who told you he is working on correcting the problem. Love it!! If this were my dream, I would define it as an active symbolic precognitive dream that gave verbal advice for current (no pun intended) and future health and well-being.

DR. BURK'S COMMENTARY

Dr. Kemper is one of those rare physicians who pays attention to her dreams, miraculously starting this practice while in medical school, where most of the intuitive processes are forced to shut down by the rigors of the left-brained curriculum. I am always amazed when I give talks for mental health professionals and do a survey of the audience asking how many of them keep dream diaries.

The positive response rate is around 10 percent, as it is not taught in most psychotherapy training programs. It is one of my dreams for this book that it will assist in restoring dreams to their rightful place in medicine, and even perhaps to the medical school curriculum.

PART SIX

*Healing Guidance Dreams
for All Illnesses*

The original structural components of the psyche are of no less
surprising a uniformity than are those of the visible body.
— CARL JUNG, *CW 11, Para 845*

This section works with healing guidance dreams that may be helpful to more illnesses than just cancer. The first three chapters were
contributed by Wanda, Kat, and Diane, who were participants in
Dr. Larry Burk's Breast Cancer Dreams Project and contributed
prophetic dreams we examined earlier. The healing dreams of
other dreamers complete this section.

37

Dream Imagery for Healing

Wanda Burch

I dreamed two important dreams before my biopsy for breast cancer, which I recounted in my book, *She Who Dreams*, and which is excerpted in this book. The cone breast presented me with the gift of learning to use the imagery from my dreams. The second dream was of equal importance. I would look at this dream over a year later and realize that it was a companion dream to a "big" dream that finally released me from the confining shadows of my dance hall dream in Chapter 13.

This dream was the real beginning of my second journey. It contained Biblical and other images, most of them unfamiliar to me. A friend assisted me in the magic of the dream.

Into the Pool of Healing

I walk with my friend to the pool at Bethesda. There is a long row of steps with a columned arcade above, and I meet an angel who says his name is Eliseus. I ask the angel for help, but no one seems to come. I hold my friend's hand, as a child would hold a hand, and I move cautiously to the edge of the pool. Another angel moves forward, perhaps the same one, and stands beside me. This angel tells me I will find healing in the "rushes" or "rushing."

I move suddenly into a village landscape, and an enormous spider appears. I do not like spiders, and I really do not like this spider. I don't know what to do about the spider, so I decide to make it less frightening. I turn it into a wind-up toy and send it away.

I move away from the now harmless spider and become a "cowherd." A large soft-eyed cow—a real cow—is looking at me. I gently place my hands on either side of her head and easily remove her head.

I move to a place where a door is being erected or re-erected among ruins, and I place it above the door. I run my hands over her head, turning it into the head of a ram.

189

I needed to understand all of the references in this dream. I went to the local library and found a 19th-century Bible with an extensive concordance. I looked up the words "Bethesda" and "Eliseus" and began with the Biblical verses themselves:

> Now there is at Jerusalem by the Sheep Market (or gate) a pool, which is called in the Hebrew tongue Bethesda, having five porches. In these lay a great multitude of impotent folk, of blind, halt, withered, waiting for the moving of the water. For an angel went down at a certain season into the pool, and troubled the water: whosoever then first after the troubling of the water stepped in was made whole of whatever disease he had.   — *John 5: 2-4*

The Pool of Bethesda was an ancient place that boasted remarkable healing powers. The name of the pool, Bethesda, was Hebrew and translated as "the house of mercy." Those who were sick or diseased came in large numbers to this pool for healing, but not all of them were healed. In the area around the pool were five porches, cloisters, piazzas, or roofed walks, described much like the arcade I had seen in my dream.

In the stories of the miraculous healings at the Pool of Bethesda, an angel of the Lord would "trouble" the water and whoever would step first into the pool after the troubling or "rushing" of the water would be healed. The wisdom of the angel would determine when the waters would be "troubled," thus determining who would be healed and who would not.

However, the responsibility for healing was shared with the person with the disease. That person had to step forward at the right moment and aggressively pursue his or her own healing. Healing, when it occurred, was instantaneous, and it was never failing in its effects.

Archeologists have investigated what they believe to be the Pool of Bethesda and believe the reference to the "season" concerns underground intermittent springs that only "rushed" into the now arid pool at intervals of several hours at specific times during the year. There is a story associated with the pool, in which a sleeping dragon, when awake, swallows or stops the water and, when asleep, allows the water to flow from its mouth back into the pool.

Other Bible verses in the book of Nehemiah (Nehemiah 2) described the rebuilding of the temple of Jerusalem and further defined the location of the Pool of Bethesda. The Pool of Bethesda was located in the Sheep Market near the temple, just to the north of the temple court. The Sheep Gate of the city was also near the temple. The Sheep Market of modern Jerusalem was not far from the general area of the ancient market. In the Nehemiah chapters were long descriptions of the families who began to rebuild the temple area, including the description of the rebuilding of the Sheep Gate near the Pool of Bethesda.

The reconstruction of the Sheep Gate provided a link to a portion of the dream I initially thought disconnected from the images of the pool and the troubling of the water—the placing of a ram's head above a door that was being re-erected. In the dream, I was not only participating in my healing by walking first into the pool as the waters were "troubled" by the angel but also by assisting in the "restoration" of the gate, which led to the "body" of the temple.

Eliseus provided another powerful image of healing. Eliseus was the Greek name of the prophet Elisha, who both prophesied and healed in the time of Elijah. He was given a special blessing and was allowed to perform miracles of healing. Both the story of the Pool of Bethesda and the information about Eliseus were previously unfamiliar to me, their unfamiliarity making their presence in my dreaming even more powerful.

Dreams such as this were antidotes to my feelings of death and dying. They offered me the possibility of healing and presented me with possibilities of cleansing that I could use for my own miracle. The spider image as one of disease had already appeared several times in my dreams and could easily be identified with the malignancy. In this dream, I had turned the harmful, poisonous spider into a harmless child's toy.

Using Dream Imagery

I had never experimented with actively using dream imagery for healing. I sat down and considered all of the possibilities for using the image of the cone breast (from the dream I described in Chapter 1), which accurately pictured the problem and the beginning of a solution. The most obvious use was meditation, but I decided to use the dream meditation in a more active manner.

I rewrote the dream content as a simple paragraph, retaining the core elements of squeezing a cone under running water and clearing it of the dark liquid. I played simple background music and recited the dream both aloud and in my mind. I recited it before I went to bed, during the day while I worked, and taped it in the car so I could see the words, a simple recall mechanism, which turned the dream into active imagery and automatically brought it to mind instantly throughout the day.

Repetition gave the dream a different kind of energy, an active intent, in which the dream played again and again in my mind. I imagined myself pulling the radiating cells back toward the mass and then taking the cone breast, cells now contained within a single mass, and squeezing the dark fluid into a bowl. I saw the actual dream as a prescription; the use of the content of the dream as medicine for healing.

I worked tirelessly in the little time I had left before the second biopsy (which became the complete surgery) to do something, as directed, about the malignant breast lump. I continued working with the first dream of the cone but added to it the powerful dream of cleansing and healing at the Pool of Bethesda. I rewrote the new dream into a meditation called "Into the Pool of Healing." I used a tape with music and recorded the music and the meditation onto a second tape, in which I recorded my voice reading the dream. I played the tape at night before I went to sleep or during the day in the car tape player as an active meditation.

Medical Choices

After the second biopsy and surgery revealed I had been living with an aggressive, fast-moving breast cancer tumor, with cells radiating in a non-massing manner, my dreams changed. They presented choices, a further exploration of alternative and natural methods, what I called a "healing cocktail." Using surgery, dreams, and active meditation with dream imagery allowed me to safely proceed, both with the brutal surgical removal of the cancer, my left breast and many lymph nodes, and the subsequent attack on the remaining cancer cells with chemotherapy.

My nights exploded with helpful dreams. In one I worked with a friend in a sophisticated classroom. We built together an elaborate energy plant, which produced both chemical and natural energy—a complementary blend that worked in complete harmony with each other. This dream gave me the option of combining dreaming energy with surgery and chemotherapy.

Killing the Bats

In the dream I walked into a large room, a bedroom, except the bed had sides like a crib (or a hospital bed). A friend, along with my family, entered the room with me. Under the bed lay a big bat. I rushed for the bat, picked it up by the head, and broke the head in my hands, then threw it down a flight of stairs, where it was impaled on a knifelike tool protruding from the wall.

I looked up. The ceiling was covered with smaller bats. I asked for help. All of us working together—my friend, my husband, and my son—began exterminating the bats with poison until the room was clear. Then I curled up peacefully in the bed and went to sleep.

When I dreamed Killing the Bats, I had been wrestling with a course of therapy suggested by my oncologist and surgeon. Both doctors felt that the best way to approach my unusually aggressive cancer was surgery, a modified radical mastectomy, followed by aggressive chemotherapy. I wanted to be able to use every resource available to me and firmly believed I could combine my dreams with the harsh treatment suggested and possibly even eliminate some of the worst of the side effects.

The dream of Killing the Bats provided me with the guidance I needed and convinced my friends and family I was on the right course. In the dream, the destruction of the first giant bat (the parent tumor) had been accomplished through surgery (the knifelike tool). The removal of the smaller bats (the radiating cells that escaped the surgery) was accomplished with chemotherapy (poison). My peaceful response after the destruction of the remaining bats with poison answered the question of whether or not to rely on my physician's suggestion of aggressive chemotherapy.

The choices, surgery, and chemotherapy stirred in a thick syrup of dreaming, a recipe for healing, stilled my fear, presented me with hope, and actively pushed me forward.

Cocktail Ingredients: Music

After my surgery, and as my chemotherapy treatments intensified, music appeared frequently in my dreams, soothing me when I was anxious, offering voices of celebration in predictions of wellness, providing tools for healing when I felt most wounded. During the harshest days of chemotherapy treatments, I took the gift of music outside the dream.

My husband, Ron, played the organ for the local church, which was located within walking distance of our home. He often practiced at the church in the evenings. I walked with him to the church. He would turn on a foyer light and lights around the organ, leaving the main body of the church in soft darkness, lit only by the glow of the organ box.

In the dark aisle of the church below the organ box, I would lie down, my eyes closed, all of my body, arms, legs, back, head, touching the floor. The organ chords vibrated the music from the top of my head to the tip of my toes, allowing my imagination to see a flow of healing imagery through my body, washing over and through every "organ," through my blood, bone, tendons, muscles, nerves, lymph system, fibers, washing and cleansing with the deep vibrating music tones serving as an active dream.

Dreaming with the Organist

One of those evenings, drifting in and out of sleep, I thought about a friend, Millie Coutant, a popular psychic in Lake George, New York, who had died several years before. She often visited me before she died and sometimes, not often, talked about me. Once, she shared her vision of me and a predicted illness and recovery; more importantly, telling me that we create our own miracles. Comforted by that memory, I drifted asleep, lost in the music and in the warmth of the quilt and thinking about Millie.

Walking the Plank

I am looking everywhere for Millie. I want to tell her I have been ill and ask her if she knows if I will live. There are dark colors in the sky, and I try to use an enormous eraser to wash them away. I am walking on a narrow plank, and several times almost slip into soft sand. A person comes up beside me and places wider boards on either side of the small boards until I have a safe place for walking. As I reach out, I realize tubes are attached to my arms and energy food is being fed into my body through the tubes.

My new dream offered guidance in my journey, a presence that would continue to make sure I had safe passage across the shifting uncertain sand, plus I was again assured my healing cocktail of spiritual and medical resources would provide healing energy.

The dream tubes looked remarkably similar to the chemotherapy tubes in the treatment facility, but the contents, the chemicals, also referred to as a "cocktail" by the oncology nurses, would become, in my imagination, conduits for healing energy, not toxins that would make me even more ill.

More Ingredients

I noticed that each time I progressed to a new place in my recovery, my dreams changed themes. They would manifest themselves in different but similar images, in dream groups that drifted into patterns night after night, bombarding me with the imagery I needed at that particular moment, providing me with a goal until I had passed successfully to the next stage of my recovery. Then my dreams would change themes again.

Following the dream of the unseen hand placing planks for my safe passage, I dreamed of:

a broken bridge that repaired itself before I crossed;

a ladder with broken rungs mended by an invisible hand so that I could safely
climb upward;
and a swinging bridge over a gorge, broken and once again repaired by an
invisible hand.

Guidance and safe passage for the upcoming journey gleaned from simple short
dreams provided imagery that was easy to use in my meditation exercises and
easy to recall in my healing prescriptions. In dreams, I also explored the use of
"imagery"—not of particular images but of the actual process. The following
was one such dream.

The Dream Library

I asked my family to help me with my research. We were on the upper floor of the
library, looking through texts on how to use imagery and also looking for images
that might assist me in my recovery. The primary focus of the dream was the
definition of the word *imagery* as the "ability of the mind to establish a path to
healing the body." The path was different for everyone, but each person needed
a clear picture combined with a clear healing goal or intent. Seeing the body as
well and whole was a viable *intent*, if none other presented itself in a dream.
I saw myself viewing my own body as a separate object; a small version of my
body separated itself and turned in a spiral so I could view it both inside and out.

This became a useful technique for checking the health of my body when a
new pain or area of discomfort presented itself. It also became a method for
checking on the progress of my healing during the chemotherapy and beyond.
If a new symptom frightened me, or if a dream scared me, I could imaginatively
view my body in its entirety and mentally spin it around. I would immediately
be calmed if I saw nothing disturbing. I created my own dictionary of images,
taken from my dreams and consciously and actively used for my personal
healing. Intent was important. If I presented my dreaming self with a problem before I fell asleep, the working-out process would take place during the
dreaming, sometimes offering a solution in the dream or tools I could use upon
waking. This process was very effective for anxiety and depression.

Even when I experienced difficulty in bringing the dream forward into the
day, the spontaneous work exacted in the night dream translated into healing
in my body in spite of me. The stated Intent, combined with the dream images,
continued to help me battle depression, doubt, and anxiety in such subtle ways
I was often unaware of the extent of the healing process in waking reality.

During the last months of the long summer of chemotherapy, all of my dreams converged in a final barrage of healing imagery. Many were small and simple, but they piled one on top of the other, and it was impossible to determine if one might be more important than another.

I was healing slowly in spirit, somewhat faster in body. In the physical healing, I suffered radical mood swings, but through it all, my dreams presented positive images and predicted in sleep a more hopeful outcome than I allowed in waking. They foretold a time when I would feel whole again. In fact, they went beyond the feeling of wellness to a time in which I would use my own experience to help other people work with their own health problems.

Renegotiating a Soul Contract

There was one dark dream that I needed to successfully navigate. As my healing progressed, I was still haunted by my long recurring dream of the dance hall that led to a door with a passage to my death.

Dreams of healing countered that dream, but a dark dream of a messenger of death came near the anniversary of my diagnosis and held me in its grip until I received an awe-inspiring dream of renegotiating my life contract. I received that dream on the eve of my 43rd birthday.

Vibrating Light Dream

I moved up a mountain on waves of vibrating light and stood—no, cringed—in blinding light, before a presence who I begged for a life extension. I was shown a contract in which I had agreed to leave in my 43rd year, but after my pathetic pleading, I was granted a life extension and woke trembling and sobbing.

I had confronted a powerful presence, confounding my ability to describe, in order to remember my soul's contract. The contract included responsibility to others and responsibility to tell my story of intuition and dreaming, combined with the careful and caring use of all the medical technology available—my healing cocktail.

> **KAT'S INTERPRETATION**
>
> If these were my dreams, I'd be as much in awe of them as Wanda is in their healing powers. Wanda learns her own dream language and uses it to understand the symbolism in her dreams. Wanda's healing dreams are steps to a healing process, with each dream seen as a building block for the entire healing process of "building a healthy life."

The dreams are filled with healing symbolism, which is both symbolic and literal, from the *Biblical Pool of Bethesda*, a symbolic place of miraculous, instantaneous healing, to *black bats*, which may symbolize disaster "hanging around" in hidden places, while *spiders* share much in common with crabs, the universal symbolism for cancer.

DR. BURK'S COMMENTARY

When I recommend Wanda's remarkable book to cancer patients, I always mention my favorite dream image: of her toxic chemotherapy turning into energy food as it flows into her body through the IV tubes. Using dream imagery for guided meditation exercises was one of the brilliant intuitive insights that allowed her to heal so efficiently and renegotiate her contract.

In the book, she also mentioned that, in reviewing her total doses of chemotherapy at the conclusion of her treatments, one of her doctors commented that she had a remarkable tolerance for maximal dosage with minimal side effects. Her dream healing experiences were literally and figuratively "Biblical" in proportion.

38

Tiny Bubbles and Fishy Chakras

Kathleen (Kat) O'Keefe-Kanavos

My pre-chemotherapy blood test, taken yesterday, shows my blood cell count is still too low for my next treatment scheduled for tomorrow. "Wait another week, get another blood test, and have the results sent to me," my Boston oncologist said.

The phone call sent me into a deep depression. Would I ever finish these treatments? Would my life ever return to normal? Whatever normal was after cancer. My chemo schedule is four treatments over a three-month period, and so far it has taken me a whole month to recover each time. This delay would push my final chemotherapy treatment back by more than a month. My blood cells must get back up to a reasonable level quickly for me to get on with my life.

During my nightly meditation, I fell asleep and had this dream.

Tiny Bubbles

My dream shifted from my nightly meditation into shimmering golden light dancing off pure white sands, clean as newly driven snow and kissed by Caribbean blue waters. The song "Tiny Bubbles" by Hawaiian singer Don Ho plays in my dreaming mind. I am in Hawaii on a sunny beach making red-and-white bubbles by dancing in the surf with a unique bubble kit.

I pull the wand through the soapy foam on the breaking waves and wave it through the breath of fresh air, which scatters the bubbles that begin as tiny as snowflakes but grow as big as giant balloons. All the colors of the rainbow slide across the surface, but the most prominent colors are hues of red and blue, which blend together to create a majestic purple. The bubbles stick to my body and absorb into my skin, nose, and ears. I realize I am asleep and having such a beautiful, lucid dream I tell myself not to wake up.

I understood the dream, and the next day told my husband I wanted to go for another blood test. This shocked him because he knows my profound dislike of needles. "I had a dream and know my blood levels are normal today," I said.

To everyone's surprise, the test revealed my blood had returned to an acceptable level for treatment, so chemotherapy was scheduled, on time, for the next day.

KAT'S INTERPRETATION

This was a lucid healing dream that used symbolism. The *bubbles* in my dream were my white blood cells being healed by circles of life formed from the ocean of spirituality, growing in the breath of life, and empowered by the *colors of the rainbow, which correlates with the chakras*, and absorbed into my body as I dance the Dance of Life on the sands of time on the beach between life and death. Dreaming of being on a *beach or shoreline* is a common dream setting for someone in crisis, and can symbolize being on the edge of life and death or an area between land's reality and oceans spirituality. *Large bodies of water* may symbolize the unconscious, our deep emotions, spirituality, and God-centered wisdom. I had an ocean full of God washing and healing my cells. Was this just a lucid dream? I don't think so. It was a healing dream, validated by blood tests the following day.

DR. BURK'S COMMENTARY

My first exposure to the use of imagery for healing in medicine came from Dr. Bernie Siegel's book, *Love, Medicine and Miracles*, in which he described patients visualizing images of their white blood cells as Pac-Men eating up their cancer cells. I like the tiny bubbles imagery that Kat used to accomplish the opposite effect of enhancing the numbers of her white cells. As a lucid dream, it had an immediate effect, similar to the way a hypnosis session might work. Robert Waggoner has described how a lucid dreamer used blue light imagery to heal warts overnight in a fashion reminiscent of healing stories from the hypnosis literature.[62]

Fine Tuned and Fishy Healing Chakras

Peter props me gently against one of the quaint gas lamp posts lining the streets of downtown Boston, removes his scarf, and wraps it twice around my balding head.

"Stay right here while I go see if the restaurant is open, then I'll come right back for you," he says, then sprints through the drifting snow and disappears into the early fading daylight of winter.

Like I have the energy to go anywhere... He realized within minutes of our walk that I was too weak after my chemotherapy of Adriamycin and Cytoxan (aka Red Death) to walk to the restaurant and back if it were closed due to the February Nor'eastern snowstorm engulfing the area.

Yes, I am in crisis. Another nausea attack creeps over my body and beads of sweat freeze in my eyebrows. I think I'm dying.

I don't even have the energy to brush the flakes off my nose or eyelashes, so they melt and slide down my face. One man, wearing only a sweater and no gloves, pushes snow off his car.

His hands are bright red. He's probably some poor schmuck transferred here from sunny California whose closest experience to a snowstorm is a snow cone. I feel compelled to warn him about yellow snow but don't have the energy for conversation. I'll need it if the snowplow comes by and covers me up before Peter gets back. It happens here to children, and especially pets tied to posts. I'll have to bark like a dog to be found.

As the gas lamps turn on, their orange reflection shimmers on the snow. The whole street is transformed into a dreamy Kinkade painting, as waves of light play off shadows that spread with every passing second. It's the same light as the beginning of my dream last night, replaying itself now in my darkest waking hour.

The sound of feet crunching on snow pulls me from the dream memory and back to my current lamppost. True to his word, Peter reappears with a devilish grin on his face. "You'll love this restaurant. It's the perfect, romantic place you wanted."

It is a lovely little spot in the basement of an old building, made cozy by red brick walls warmed by the light of tiny white votives on blue-and-white-checkered tablecloths. Delicious aromas precede steaming plates of food. I don't eat much, but it is well worth the hiccups that follow, my early warning sign for nausea.

We celebrate my halfway point with a shared glass of red wine—shared because, with all the other "stuff" in me, especially the Ativan, drinking a glass by myself would knock me on the floor. (Maybe I should do that before my next blood test—couldn't hurt.)

"I couldn't believe how fast your blood levels recovered from Monday," Peter said, giving my hand an affectionate squeeze.

Later that night, my spirit guides join in the celebration. In a dream, they give me symbols for my chakras, a fine tuning with a fork, a flower, and my color and number.

Healing Through Chakra Meditation

Every morning, evening and often at naptime, I do my visualization and meditation, during which I often fall asleep from treatment fatigue. Truth be told, I can fall asleep standing against a wall.

However, on this particular occasion, my Franciscan monk-spirit guides appeared during meditation and led me through a pop-up window that became a Sacred Dream Doorway, behind which is a wealth of information, in a place where miracles and magic are the norms.

During the dream, spirit guides gave me colors to visualize with each chakra, and the location of the chakra was different from anything in books. Maybe this deviation from the norm was just for me, because I am not in the norm of life; I am in a fight to the death.

Healing Colors for Chakras

While concentrating on my breathing, I am transported to my special place, on a free-floating temple high in the sky, overlooking the ocean on one side and a rainforest on the other. A river runs through the forest to the ocean.

It is a calm, beautiful, round, marble platform, without walls or a ceiling, making it open to the breezes, and it is ringed with seven Greek columns and a north-facing altar. In the center of the platform is a king-size bed, surrounded by a sunken, crystal-clear freshwater aquarium filled with ancient Koi goldfish with chakra-colored fin patterns. Their flowing fins shimmer like gold as they swim around my bed.

I often sit on the edge of the platform, feet dangling in the breezes, and listen to the sounds of animals, birds, and life, as it drifts up from the forest and ocean below. It is here I do much of my thinking and work through life's challenges. Clouds act as pathways often traveled by spiritual guides who wave as they pass or come to visit. My monk guide appears. I am suddenly meditating on my dream bed.

In my meditation, I ask God to send his healing, liquid, golden light of health and love into the crown of my head and down into my chakras, where it is caught by crystal chalices. Light surrounds me like a waterfall.

Feeling my violet seventh chakra of higher spirit fill with warm liquid light, I ask the light to fill the crystal chalice housed within the chakra until it overflows into my sixth, blue chakra, located between my eyes, which stores the psychic gifts I use to access my spirit guides.

After the warmth fills my sixth chakra, it overflows into my fifth, purple, throat chakra, used for communication, until that chalice overflows into my fourth, green and pink chakra of my breasts, love, and relationships. While I am thanking God for filling this fourth cup, it overflows and completely fills both of my breasts before flowing down to my hands.

Tiny little dark spots of negativity that look like ashes wash out of my fingertips and flow into the purple flame of Saint Germain beside the bed where the negativity is converted into positive energy and returned to the universe in the form of sparks that look like tiny shooting stars.

Next, the golden liquid flows into my stomach, abdomen, pancreas, gallbladder, liver, spleen, kidneys, ovaries, uterus, and bladder, then is washed through my third, red chakra of forgiveness. The monk says, "Forgiveness is freedom from the past to heal the present in order to move into the future." Again, any negativity is cleansed by the purple flame of Saint Germain and returned to the universe.

Warm light flows down my legs to my knees, which house my second, orange chakra. I claim this as my personal chakra because, in a previous dream I titled "Color and Number" in my dream journal, I was given the number 2 as my power number and the color orange as my power color. I visualize all the people who constitute my inner self and were written about in *Surviving Cancerland* being washed with this healing light. As it flows over us and down my legs to my first chakra, my yellow, tribe chakra, I imagine the light connecting to all my tribes, both here on the earth plane and those on the other side of life—the dead.

Finally, the golden light flows out through the soles of my feet and connects me to the earth plane. Golden light flows from the top of my head, through my body, and out the soles of my feet. I can feel the healing warmth surge through my body, causing me to perspire.

The dream shifts, and I am lying on my stomach on a massage table, unable to remember how I got here. A bright angel gowned in white appears next to me with a tuning fork, which she strikes on her hand to create a perfect tone, then passes the vibrating fork and sound over my aura, body, and spine. I become one with the sound, and my body vibrates in harmony with the perfection of this God-tone, causing the bed to vibrate, which awakens me.

Lying perfectly still, I close my eyes and reenter my previous dream-state and discover I am still pulsating like crazy on the massage table and wonder if I should wake up again.

A voice in my mind says, "Wait."

All the crystal chalices from my previous dream on my dream-bed reappear and combine to become one large goblet brilliant with all the transparent colors of my chakras. It glows like a giant diamond as it fills with golden liquid light.

"Drink, in the name of the Father, Son, and Holy Spirit," the voice says.

Okay, I think and drink the warm liquid in my mind. Is that all?

"Lift up a portion of your skin on your arm and look under it," the voice commands.

In my dream, I lift up a flap of skin and see the bright golden light glowing from deep within my arm.

Another voice says, "She's really cookin' now!"

Is that all, now? I ask the voices in my mind, again.

"Wait."

Two angels appear on either side of me and begin to brush off my body and aura with fans made of three large white feathers. Next, my monk-spirit guide places ancient-looking symbols on translucent triangles of swordfish. The symbols are different from anything I have ever seen in books. Each triangle and symbol becomes saturated with the chakra color and pulsates with God-vibration. The pulsating fish triangles with symbols are placed on my chakras. *Am I done, now?* I ask the voice a third time.

"Sleep," the voice answers gently, and a hand extends from time and space, much like the hand seen on the Ace of Wands tarot card, to hand me a beautiful yellow dandelion.

"This is your flower. Use it as a wand to touch anything you wish to change. Keep it safe in your heart chakra for whenever you need it."

I awoke the next morning refreshed and dressed for the long drive into Boston for my last chemotherapy treatment.

KAT'S INTERPRETATION

The dream is literal, symbolic, and lucid because the dreamer knew she was dreaming and was able to exit and reenter the dream. It was also a healing dream, because it showed spiritual and physical healing in progress, later validated by medical tests in the form of pre- and post-dream blood tests.

This dream is so complex that pages of interpretation might not do justice to uncovering its meanings, messages, signs, and symbols, so please feel free to expand on it in your dream journal or dream circles.

Chapter 5 in this book discusses dream types. However, some dreams can overlap with others. Even in guided dreams filled with conversation, there may be symbolism, a play on words, or dualities.

Dualities are two elements in a dream that have a concealed form in symbolism and a revealed form in the obvious. For instance, an ocean can be a "body of water" but also the Spiritual Body of God, or consciousness. This lucid healing dream is filled with dualities that give balance to heaven and earth and has a play on words, as in "sole of the feet," or soul. Numerology plays a significant role in dream interpretation. The dream contains three circles within circles: the circular platform, Greek columns, and the aquarium around the bed. The *number 2* is given as a sacred number and appears throughout the dream (2 is the number for duality and balance and symbolizes choice).

A triangle has *three* sides, and in a dream can denote a connection to the spiritual realm. In Christianity and Judaism, a triangle is a symbol for God. The *number 3* is also symbolic of mind, body, spirit; the Trinity; and the id, ego, and superego, and is considered an angel number and magical. This dream contains inner selves, spirituality, and angels intent on helping to heal the dreamer.

Swordfish is a juxtaposed play on words. *Swords* symbolize "battle," and *fish* is the "Christ symbol," so the meaning may be going to war armed with Christ.

Sound therapy is a means of healing in many ancient cultures, and in the dream, it can represent the duality of sound therapy or being in tune with life while being healed with a note of perfection.

Dandelion is also a duality and play on words: a dandy lion. Dandelion translates to *dent-de-lion* in French, which means "the lion's tooth." In a dream, it reflects courage, pride, and family communication. In the world of natural medicine, dandelion is used for detoxing the body. The spiritual meaning has been linked with Christ's self-sacrifice on the cross, as depicted in art from the Netherlands that shows the dandelion in crucifixion paintings. Yellow is symbolic of communication, clarity, and associated with the healing power of the sun, quick wit, and alertness of thought for problem-solving. In the dream, it is given as a wand for powerful transformation.

DR. BURK'S COMMENTARY

Wow, hard to imagine what it must have been like to have had this dream. Kat points out that her meditations sometimes morph into dreams, and it is clear that there is a broad spectrum of altered states of consciousness available to us for healing, from meditation to visualization to dreaming to lucidity to out-of-body experiences, and beyond.

Of course, it is a special bonus to have participation by monks and angels, if those kinds of magical guides are available to you. If not, focusing directly on breathing, colors, and the chakras is a good place to start your healing process.

39

The Raw Food Diet Dream

Diane

I had a lumpectomy after my diagnostic precognitive dream and wasn't certain what other types of therapies I wanted to pursue, as described in Dr. Larry Burk's book *Let Magic Happen*.[63] I pondered strong advice from my doctors to undergo chemotherapy and radiation and consulted with several holistic oncologists, who all told me to do the standard treatments.

But then I started having dreams of a different raw vegetable every night.

Green Beans

In the dream, green beans are hanging on a clothesline, gently blowing in the breeze.

Rabbi

I went to a teaching session with a rabbi. As each person before me walked in, the rabbi gave them a prayer book. When I came in, he handed me a large bowl of fresh green vegetables.

As it turns out, in real time, about a month after the second dream, I went on a retreat with that rabbi. When he found out I had breast cancer, he put his hand on my head to bless me. After a few moments of silence, he said to me, "If you can do wheatgrass it would be good for you."

That did it!

I agreed to take a short course of Tamoxifen, but also did research on raw vegetarian diets. I discovered the Hippocrates Health Institute in Florida and went on their raw food diet for one year, and have since developed mindfulness retreats for women touched by cancer, which of course involve mindful eating.

KAT'S INTERPRETATION

If this were my dream, I would define it as a diagnostic, healing, and precognitive, because the rabbi in her dream who handed her a bowl of vegetables was again met in the waking world, where he told her "wheatgrass would be good for you." It is also symbolic, because the vegetables were hanging on a clothesline, which may be symbolic of dry vegetables being a good choice as well. The mental image of plants hanging and flapping in the breeze is a difficult one to forget, which reinforces the idea mentioned earlier in the book: the stranger the dream, the more important the message.

DR. BURK'S COMMENTARY

With Diane's initial experience of having a vivid precognitive diagnostic dream, it is little surprise that she would have another very direct one to guide her dietary healing journey. Precognitive dreams have a way of getting your attention like almost nothing else, other than perhaps a near-death experience without the actual physical trauma. It allowed her the confidence to forego the conventional radiation and chemotherapy and to follow her intuition. Nutritional therapies for cancer vary widely, from macrobiotic approaches to ketogenic diets, so tailoring it to the individual is of particular importance. What better way than directly from your own dreams?

40

Silver Spaceship Aliens Saved My Life

Dana Anderson

This story originally appeared in Chapter 3 of The Meaning of Dreaming *by Savitri Simpson (Crystal Clarity Publishers, 2016).*

At age 29, as a single mom with a two-year-old-daughter, I was diagnosed with stage 4 uterine cancer. Although I was going through chemotherapy and all the usual procedures to try to save my life, the prognosis was not good. In fact, I had a 5 percent chance of surviving!

Nevertheless, I was determined to live and to be able to raise my daughter and pursued every possible means of healing.

In the midst all of this, I had a dream that did, I truly believe, save my life.

The Silver Saucer Spaceship

In the dream, aliens landed in a silver saucer spaceship. They approached me and told me, "What you need is called Interferon." Then they handed me some.

I had no idea what Interferon was! But the message was so clear and the word so distinct. I had worked with dreams enough to recognize aliens as a metaphor for "information coming from above and beyond." Because the message was so vivid and precise, I told my doctor about the dream.

He was silent for a moment and then said that Interferon was a new type of treatment, currently still being tested. He was very struck by the fact that I had dreamed this very unusual and particular word. On that basis, he wrote me a prescription for Interferon, which acts to boost the white blood cells of the immune system.

This was one of several specific healing dreams I had that directed me in my process of full and complete healing from stage 4 uterine cancer. The cancer went into full remission and remains that way to date, 18 years later.

I know these were divine messages from God and my healing was a complete miracle and grace. To this day I am grateful to be alive.

KAT'S INTERPRETATION

Dana Anderson was well versed in her own dream language and understood the message in the dream. Healing dreams can happen during treatment to change the course of therapy from one of "the norm" to one of success. If this were my dream, I would define the dream as literal, because Dana heard conversation from the aliens, who gave her the name of a particular medication that she was unfamiliar with that that her doctor immediately recognized as new for uterine cancer.

DR. BURK'S COMMENTARY

Interferon is a type of cytokine, proteins made by cells in response to tumor cells. It can be made as a drug through recombinant gene technology, and it is administered along with chemotherapy regimens. That Dana would be able to dream specifically of such a high-tech therapy is quite remarkable. For her to survive stage 4 cancer puts her into the category of radical remission discussed earlier in Chapter 10. She is indeed fortunate that her doctor was impressed by her dream guidance and followed through on it.

41

Bliss behind the Mask of Addiction

Deborah O'Brien

I've never been a big visual dreamer (dreams with pictures) but have always had dream auditory messages. I hear strong life-saving messages in my sleep. Sometimes, it is just my name—*Debbie*—drawn out, to wake me. And before awakening, I would say, "Oh, there's that voice in my dream."

From the day my mother gave birth to me, she was never well enough to care for me because her placenta ripped. I was born with a mask of placenta on my face, called a caul. My very superstitious aunt from Ireland said it was either a sign of evil or a blessing. Mom became pernicious anemic, which always made me feel guilty. I missed bonding with Mom. It was the beginning of my life behind a mask that killed me and then dreamed me back to a new life.

On Memorial Day, 1991, my son was flown home from the first Persian Gulf War by the Red Cross and taken to Massachusetts General Hospital to join his four siblings to say goodbye to me, his mother. At age 45, the poison from excessive drug and alcohol abuse was in my bloodstream.

I Was Dying

Despite the valiant efforts of a team of doctors, who put me on a blood-filtering machine and fed me charcoal brackets to keep me from vomiting, I got worse. Four huge men in white coats shackled my wrists and ankles as my tiny tremors turned into violent convolutions. When a lung collapsed, my organs started to shut down, and I had a heart attack.

My Uncle, Father Bill, Gave Me Last Rites.

The voice in my mind said, *Look at what you have done to your children. Look at how you have made them suffer. You are such a loser. You can't do anything right.*

I could not listen to the voice torment me anymore because it was right. So I closed my eyes and quietly slipped away.

Six days later, on my birthday, I awoke, reborn, from a dream, but didn't know it yet.

Feeling awake, I found myself all alone in a very bright and extremely clean room. It felt like I was lying on a cold, hard table instead of a nice, warm bed.

Am I dead? Maybe I am in the morgue, I wondered. But I didn't *feel* dead... as if I knew what that felt like. Then I thought I must be in the operating room. It certainly was a sterile room. Then I wondered if I was really awake.

All of a sudden I felt very tired, and it was getting too hard to think. While I lay there on the cold, hard table, I wanted to pray, but could not. My mind would not cooperate. I could neither pray to live nor pray to die. I wanted God to decide. The only thought I could formulate was, "Thy will be done." Like a broken record, these four words repeated in my head.

The soothing rhythm of my breath going in and going out helped calm me. Then there was silence. A beautiful sense of serenity fell over me like a warm blanket. It was in this stillness I surrendered. "Thy will be done. . ."

In the space of nothingness, my mind could not dwell on the past or the future, and it was unable to torment me with its vindictive alcoholic voice. "Thy will be done... "

In this state of hallucinogenic dreaming, I could only feel.

A Tingling Dream

At first, I felt a tiny tingling in my feet and hands. As the vibration pulsated stronger, I felt a flutter in my stomach, which became an intense throbbing in my groin, my first chakra. It moved into my abdomen, my second chakra, then all the way up into my heart chakra. I was coming back to life. It felt like something was swelling up inside me. The vibration in my heart felt like my heart would burst as it overflowed with a sensation of gratitude like I had never experienced before. It felt like I could not contain the feeling, like it was going to pour out of me, right through each and every one of my pores. Then I felt bliss.

Suddenly, I was engulfed in God's pure light. It was radiating through every inch of my being, down into my cells. As the white light washed over me, I felt like I was bathed in its loving frequency. I felt so clean, warm, and reborn.

Lying there, surrendered in God's presence, I felt His unconditional love, His amazing grace, and His peace.

I didn't die. I came alive! And woke up. Lying there, awake in God's pure light, I felt like He had washed all my sins away. Then I felt His peace. His peace *did* "surpass all understanding." There is nothing else in this world like the feeling of God's peace.

When I started meditating, I was surprised to have the same beautiful breathing and healing experience again. You can have it too. The peace of God is inside all of us. It's the peace Jesus promised. It's the freedom you dream about.

Since that fateful time, 26 years ago, I have not touched a drop of liquor or any drugs. My desire for them dissolved like a nightmare caught in the morning sun. My dream healed me.

Peace I leave you, my peace I give you; not as the world gives it do I give it to you. Let not your heart be troubled, nor let it be afraid (John 14:27).

KAT'S INTERPRETATION

If this were my dream I would consider it a hypnogogic healing dream, which can leave the dreamer wondering if they are awake or asleep and often feels hallucinogenic in nature.

DR. BURK'S COMMENTARY

It sounds like what Deborah has described was a near-death experience (NDE) in dream form, leading to her literal resurrection from addiction. The description of energy moving through the chakras is also typical of a *kundalini* process, which may result in immersion in the divine white light. It certainly was no ordinary dream, as I doubt that even a vivid precognitive dream like those reported in the Breast Cancer Research Project could have cured alcoholism. However, NDEs typically have four transformative aspects, including loss of fear of death, a sense of life purpose, enhanced psychic abilities, and altered electrophysiology, all of which may have contributed to her healing.[64]

42

Cystic Fibrosis/Organ Transplant: Life from the Edge of Death

Inka Nisinbaum

After my birth in 1979, doctors told my parents I had only four years to live because I was born with cystic fibrosis, a genetic disease inherited from your parents that affects your lungs, digestive system, and liver. It isn't curable and will eventually kill you, earlier rather than later.

At the time, no one knew much about cystic fibrosis, CF for short. The prognosis devastated my parents. Yet, I grew up, thanks to many pills, intravenous antibiotic therapies, and running. Running kept my lungs clean, kept me ahead of CF, and made me resilient.

Twenty-two years later, while studying psychology and preparing to enter my next phase of life, my CF suddenly caught up with me.

One morning in March, on my way to the university, I realized this was not the life I wanted to live anymore. Due to my failing liver, my abdomen was filled with liquid, extremely painful, and ridiculously swollen. I looked like I was eight months pregnant. I struggled for each breath. My fight against the disease was lost.

On April 2, 2001, I accepted the fact that a double lung and liver organ transplant was my only chance to survive. But tragedy struck when a dear friend of mine, Mario, died in a motorcycle accident. It was like our souls knew each other more than we did. I didn't have much time to mourn him because a few days later, I was having a hernia operation and struggling to recover. My time of running had shifted to struggling—struggling with recovery and struggling with life. There was no space for anyone besides myself, so I forgot about Mario.

On September 11, 2001, (9/11) I received a letter officially listing me for a double lung and liver transplant. This day symbolized a new beginning for me. From that day on, my struggling shared space with waiting for the phone call saying my clinic received organs for me. On August 18, 2001, I got a welcomed visitor in a dream.

Mario Is With Me

Mario, the dead friend I hadn't thought of for so many months, or get a chance to say a proper goodbye to, stopped by in my dream. We were sitting in a house in the living room, just talking as we always did, while there was a lot of activity around us. It appeared as though someone was moving in or out, but I wasn't sure. And while we talked, I couldn't help but wonder why Mario was here in my dream, sitting right next to me, while being dead.

The moment I started to wake up, I knew Mario was dead, of course, but still here with me and would protect and take care of me during the transplant. This feeling was so clear and real, I immediately wrote down my dream.

On January 22, 2002, I had another dream showing me I was taken care of and had nothing to worry about.

I dreamed I was in the hospital, waking up completely surprised that my triple organ transplant had not been a big deal after all. The whole operation took four hours, I didn't have any pain, and I was able to stand up. My legs were a little swollen, but that passed very quickly. I went up and down the hall and could actually breathe. But I wasn't ready to look at my belly yet and afraid to touch the fresh scars. Still, my transplant was a walk in the park; so perfect that I had forgotten to tell everyone about it. Nobody knew I was in the hospital, getting new organs.

I wrote, "Last night I had an absolutely cool dream." Another moment of hope, another moment of gratitude, and another moment I was able to believe in what I wished for—a healthy life past my transplant. Eventually, I had to wait 15 months for my transplant. My dreams were bloody and brutal during this time, symbolizing my inner fight. But on December 28, 2002, three days after Christmas, the call came: my transplant clinic had organs waiting for me.

The transplant itself went as well as you can hope for when you get lungs and a liver replaced. While recovering in ICU, nurses sedated me for seven days, and I dreamed a lot. One reoccurring dream was extraordinary and always had the same scenery.

The Face of Death?

It was a dark night on an empty street in the city. It had rained, the streets were still wet, and the light of the streetlights reflected on the puddles. I stood on the street alone, not sure what I was supposed to do or why I was there, when

I spotted a telephone booth. In it was a man standing in a long coat and a hat, beige fabric reminiscent of 1960s attire. Every time I spotted him, he half-turned, opened the door of the telephone booth, and started to walk down the street. Every time I saw him taking off, I knew as long as I could see him, as long as I didn't lose him, as long as he didn't turn around and show me his face, I was safe.

After I was able to talk, I told my mom about this dream, and she knew immediately who the man was. It was my uncle, her brother. He always wore long coats and hats in beige. I had never met my uncle, because he died from Hodgkin's lymphoma, at the age of 37, 10 days before my birth. He never said "hi" again in any of my dreams after I was released from the hospital, but because he was there for me when I needed him the most, I feel close to him. I'm sure he will be the one picking me up once my time has come. Something I look forward to.

After 10 days, I moved to a regular hospital bed, but the nights still scared me. My dreams were filled with people all the time. It was like everyone I ever ran into came to visit me in my dreams. People I knew, people I loved, but also people I hadn't thought of in years. They all came by, but didn't say anything; they were just there, overcrowding my dreams. Finally, I requested sleeping pills to sleep deeper, to avoid all the people.

Looking back, my dreams made it look a little too easy recovering from an organ transplant. I am healthy now and even made the impossible possible by becoming a mother in 2013. I'm the only woman worldwide who had a baby after a double lung and liver transplant. I always said that God had sent me back, but forgot to tell me what I'm supposed to do here. Getting back to health was a road with many obstacles and many steps backward, but eventually, the prediction of my dreams did come true.

In 2005, I met my future husband, a man who is giving me all the support I need in order to believe in my life, myself, and my health. I had dreamed a brutal dream every week, but now I dream two per year. My fighting is over. I'm healthy now, as are my dreams, just as they predicted.

KAT'S INTERPRETATION

If these were my dreams, as is the case of many of the dreamers in this book of dreams that came true and saved lives, I would define them as multiple precognitive dreams showing her a successful surgery, lucid healing dreams within dream visitations by dead loved ones. These dreams were an important part of Inka's dreamwork journey to a healthy life.

Dreams that lead to other dreams with visitations from families and friends (often to the point of distraction) are like energizing breadcrumbs (mana from heaven) the dreamer follows and consumes as the next healing step.

Inka's first dream of Mario was a lucid dream, because she wondered why she was sitting with him in her *dream living room* when she knew he was dead. A *house* can represent a physical body, and a living room is a play on words—the room in which you live, the heart of your home. Inka's second dream was a precognitive dream, showing her future with a successful operation—she would live. The validation for that dream was her successful multi-organ transplant, a child, and a loving husband.

Inka's third dream was recurrent, because she had it many times when she was in ICU and knew that if she did not see the man's face, she would live. Dreams that take place *during the night* or are dark are often shamanic healing dreams. *Rain/water* is spirituality and indicative of emotions and emotional states. It may also suggest purifying and renewal. Inka was in critical condition in the realm between realms, where the dead can visit, and the living can wait. The *phone booth* is often seen in dreams and may represent the desire to contact someone. The validation for this dream was Inka's mother recognizing her dead brother, who had died before Inka was born.

DR. BURK'S COMMENTARY

When I was in medical school in the 1970s, most patients with cystic fibrosis rarely made it out of their teens. Mutations in the gene for the transmembrane conductance regulator protein result in marked thickening of secretions, leading to chronic lung infections. More modern treatments have extended their life expectancy, and now with the availability of organ transplants, many of the organs damaged by the genetic disease can be replaced, as in Inka's case.

The modern era of transplantation began in the 1980s during my residency, and it was initially a Wild, Wild West of medical heroics, with blood-bath liver surgeries lasting the better part of a day and a night. It is much more routine these days, with multiple organs transplanted in a single efficient surgery, but still a considerable ordeal—much more arduous than implied by her second encouraging but inaccurate dream.

Perhaps the overly optimistic dream was what she needed to get her through the intense week of sedation in the ICU and lengthy recovery afterward. Having her friend Mario and uncle as guides seemed to give her the confidence to carry on and eventually accomplish the remarkable feat of giving birth years later. As a side note, there are numerous reports of organ transplant recipients, particularly heart transplants, having dreams related to their deceased donors.

I wonder if the donors are still watching over their organs to make sure their donations are not in vain. Inka's story of a childhood illness guided to resolution through adult dreams leads into Part Seven, which begins with a child's healing dream.

PART SEVEN

Children's Dreams

43

"Up, Up, Up!"

Kathi Kemper MD, MPH

While doing my pediatric residency training at the University of Wisconsin, one of my tasks was to do a daily physical examination of each child who had undergone bone marrow transplantation (usually for cancer). Needless to say, most children do not like to awaken early in the morning in the hospital for a physical exam and blood draw. One morning, one of the little girls was already up and incredibly cheerful.

"What's going on?" I asked. "You sure are in a good mood today."

She answered confidently, "That's because my (blood) count is going up today!"

"That would be great, but we usually wouldn't expect to see the blood counts rise for another day or two," I responded cautiously. "Why do you think they'll go up today?"

She explained, "I had a dream last night that the thermometer was going up, up, up, and that means my blood count is going up."

Curious, we did the exam and sent her blood test off as usual.

Indeed, her blood counts had dramatically increased, days before expected.

That has made me respect patients' dreams and pay attention to their clues. It could have meant she would develop a fever—after all, it was a thermometer going up, but she interpreted her own dream accurately.

KAT'S INTERPRETATION

If this were my dream, I would consider it a symbolic precognitive diagnostic healing dream, with the symbolism of the thermometer being "her levels" rising that have not yet been seen. The dream was showing a healing taking place that would be validated in the future by medical tests. This child understood the positive aspect of her dream and was confident enough in it to share it with her doctor.

DR. BURK'S COMMENTARY

This dream reminds me of Kat's "Tiny Bubbles" dream. Of course, it can't be determined whether the dream itself was the cause of the blood count going up, as in Kat's case, or was actually a precognitive dream predicting the result of the test the next day. Interesting that the child was able to confidently interpret it in a positive way, despite the other possible negative interpretation with regard to the development of a fever. It is a principle of the IASD approach to dream interpretation that the dreamer always has the final word. This remarkable dream, reported by a holistic pediatrician, is a perfect transition to the following chapter by holistic surgeon Dr. Bernie Siegel about children's dreams.

44

Psyche, Soma, Healing, and Collective Consciousness

Bernie Siegel, MD

They are short, clear, coherent, easy to understand,
unambiguous, and yet unquestionable dreams.
— **SIGMUND FREUD** *Dreams of Childhood, 1920*

What presents in a dream to a child can be related to a child's physical experiences, as well as their psychological and spiritual status and nature. Their open-mindedness is a pleasure to work with because they do not fear that their dreams will not be correct, as adults do. I have had many adults refuse my help because they are not artists or handed me a page of instructions on how to draw a dream I asked them to draw. Adults are so busy thinking that they lose their minds, literally. The wisdom of the dream and consciousness is not available to them because they do not connect with their feelings and intuitive knowledge.

Dreams are creations, and creation is a miracle, so join in, and let the infinite mind and voice speak to you, and through you, to the children of the world. Young children's brains have a brainwave pattern similar to that of hypnotized individuals. Their brains are like a blank canvas upon which abusive or healing works of art can be created and made visual.

One of our children filled a canvas with the word, "words." You will notice, as I did, that "wordswordswords" become "swordswordswords," and as a surgeon he made me realize that words can both kill or cure someone. Our image of the words is the result of our responding to the image within our consciousness. I was a pediatric surgeon and realized how powerful my words were to the children who had faith in me and their parents. My words became their images and truth. Telling children that they would go to sleep in the operating room, as I was thinking about anesthesia, led them to fall asleep when we wheeled them into the operating room. They took my words literally, and it changed their picture. Just as telling them an alcohol sponge would numb their skin and they would not feel the needle.

Children are open to experiencing and believing in dreams because they have not been taught to believe their authority figures or to feel embarrassed about sharing their unique experiences. Messages from angels and deceased loved ones in dreams are all real to them, as they are to me also, because I have experienced them all, and therefore, cannot and do not deny the truth.

I had a near-death experience as a four-year-old choking on a toy, which put me into a dreamlike state. I was home in bed with one of my frequent ear infections. I took a toy telephone I was playing with, unscrewed the dial, and put all the pieces in my mouth, as I had seen carpenters do with nails, which they then pulled out to use. The problem was that I aspirated the pieces and went into laryngospasm. I can still feel my intercostal muscles and diaphragm contracting forcefully, trying to get some air into my lungs, but nothing worked, and I was unable to make any sounds to attract help. I had no sense of time but suddenly realized I was not struggling anymore. I was now above the head of the bed, watching my body dying. My self was now free of the body I had been in.

I found it fascinating to be free of my body, and a blessing. I interpret that as revealing that consciousness and body, psyche, and soma are two distinct entities. I never stopped to think about how I could still see and think while out of my body. I was feeling sorry that my mother, who was in the kitchen, would find me dead, but I thought it over and found my new state preferable and intellectually chose death over life, as do most children who experience this.

Then the boy on the bed, whom I no longer did identified as me, had an agonal seizure, vomited, and all the toy pieces came flying out. He began to breathe again, and I was very angry when I returned to my body against my will, as if I were sucked up by a vacuum cleaner. I can still remember yelling, "Who did that?" My thought as a four-year-old was that there was a God who had a schedule, and I wasn't supposed to die now. My angel apparently did a Heimlich maneuver on me is how I would explain it today.

As a result of my later life experiences, I really do believe that there is a schedule we create and are aware of unconsciously. Twice, I have had my car totaled by people driving through red lights, and once I fell off our roof when the top rung on my wooden ladder snapped off. In none of these incidents did any significant injury occur to my body.

Someone told me it was because I had an angel and he knew his name. I asked what it was, and he asked, "What did you say when the ladder broke?"

"I said, Oh, shit!"

He said, "That's his name."

I will add that I started laughing, and he always shows up when I call him in an impassioned way.

We all need to share these experiences and the resources that dreams provide us with, rather than worry what other people will think about us and our experiences. A dream is a picture created in our mind. By keeping a journal of dream drawings, you can discover the same thing that a written dream diary will reveal to you. Using art as a form of dream journaling can be helpful to children and adults who lack the vocabulary to describe a dream. Again, the image presents the facts and can be interpreted more easily than some symbolic dream meaning.

Dreams and Drawing a Tumor

At age seven, one of our kids told me his knee hurt and he needed an X-ray. I told him a hot bath seemed more appropriate. But he insisted, and because of my experience with inner wisdom we did an X-ray—and no coincidence, it revealed a tumor. I assumed it was malignant and was very depressed until the day after his X-ray, when he became my therapist and told me I was handling this poorly. The surgery revealed a rare benign tumor, and he is fine today.

In terms of drawings revealing dream material and the truth, many children make the connection. One child, who had never seen the operating room she was to enter, drew a picture of it before surgery. Symbolically, she revealed the two lights and four black knobs on the lights, the colored drapes she would be covered with, and that four people would be caring for her, all of which were correct.

Dreams reveal past, present, and future. When someone dreams and then draws the devil giving them poison or the operating room as an empty black box, they are in for trouble if they do not alter their beliefs. Through imagery, we can reprogram our minds and bodies by seeing the same things as successful and healing. So if you have choices about whom to marry, which job to take, where to live or go to college, draw your dream and the options, and you will see their benefits and problems and the best choice for you.

For adults, I have this advice: stop worrying about the fact that you are not an artist. Dreams and drawings do not need an artist to portray the truth. I have had parents with an illness have their child draw their picture for them. Could the child have dreamed for another, as seen in Part Eight of this book, as the ancient Egyptians and Greeks believed possible, and then drawn that dream for the parent? Of course, the child intuitively reveals the truth, but fear should not stop you from helping yourself and showing your inner wisdom.

One child drew a purple balloon draped in black at the top of the page, with her name on the balloon. Around it were colorful dots. I told the mom that her daughter was ready to go and to take her home and love her.

I said I didn't know what the colorful dots meant, but I learned when her mom called to say, "Bernie, Amber woke up today, my birthday, and said, 'Mom, I'm dying today as a gift to you, to free you from all the trouble.'" When we counted the dots, we realized they represented the days left in her life. Amber had dreamed her end of life and shared it as a drawing with her parents.

Daydreams and Visualization

A young boy with a brain tumor kept visualizing a fighter plane flying around in his skull and blasting the tumor. He was too sick to attend school at the time. One day, he told his parents there was no longer any tumor, just a white spot. He improved physically, and his parents allowed him to return to school. A few weeks later he fell in the gym and hit his head. A scan was done, and all that was seen was a small calcification. No tumor—just a white spot.

A boy with no palpable testicles came to the operating room with his drawing of himself. The question was, "Did he have any testicles?" His picture showed him with very long legs, and he handed it to me and said, "They're too high up." Case solved.

A girl and her mother came to my office, and the mother said, "My daughter has large lymph nodes in her neck. Lymphoma is in our family, and I am afraid she has it." The mother handed me two drawings. One was the child with her swollen face and neck, and the other was a large cat with very prominent claws. I said to the mother, "Don't worry she has cat-scratch fever." Her biopsy revealed it to be the diagnosis. Many of these drawings are displayed in my book, *The Art of Healing.*

Another child was given a coloring book that the anesthesiologist, having seen the beneficial effects of children's drawings, had made for children to fill in before surgery. It said on the first page that the anesthesiologist would be wearing what looks like green pajamas, but the child drew him in red. When I pointed this out, the anesthesiologist said that the child's mother has muscular dystrophy and he could have genes that meant he could be adversely affected by muscle relaxants, thereby threatening his life. I said to look at the last page of the book, which shows a child going home with his mom, and if he drew himself in purple, a spiritual color signifying his death, the surgery would be canceled. The last page showed him in red and black, hurting and not happy but alive, so on we went.

One family with six members came in. One of their children had cancer and said, "I don't get enough time from my family."

I didn't discuss everyone's schedule; I just said, "Draw a picture of your family."

She handed me a drawing in which everyone was on the sofa with one seat empty, and she was sitting by herself, alone on a chair. This impacted the parents, and they went home with a very different schedule of planned family participation for their daughter.

If the dream experiences of children do not make me a believer about the collective consciousness, nothing will. I totally believe that consciousness is nonlocal and not limited to the body. I also have experienced this through the drawings and dreams of patients I have cared for, which allows them to know their diagnosis and what the future holds for them.

As Jung said, "The future is unconsciously prepared long in advance and therefore can be guessed by clairvoyants," as we shall see in Part Eight, where our dreamers tune in to the illnesses of other people.

PART EIGHT

Dreams for Diagnosis of
Other People's Cancers and Illnesses –
Dreaming with and for Others

Now, since the psychic process, like any other life-process, is not just a
causal sequence, but is also a process with a teleological orientation,
we might expect dreams to give us certain indicia about the objective
causality as well as about the objective tendencies, because
they are nothing less than self-portraits of the psychic life-process.
~ **CARL JUNG,** *CW 7, Para 210*

Dreaming with and for others is a phenomenon that has been recorded and celebrated since ancient Egyptian and Greek times. It includes tandem dreaming, wherein dreamers share or enter each other's dreams simultaneously during the night. In this section, we look at how dreams are able to connect us to other dreamers, using Universal Oneness. Perhaps we are, indeed, our brothers' and sisters' keepers.

45

Kidney and Lung Cancers

Larry Burk, MD, CEHP

My very first personal experience of dream diagnosis came in 1987 on Thanksgiving evening after dinner with my parents who were visiting me in Philadelphia.

> I dreamt that I had a tumor on the left side of my brain on a CT scan. Everyone was shocked because I looked so healthy.

It was the first dream of cancer in my life, but I just wrote it down in my dream diary and didn't think anything more about it. A week later, I was at the Radiological Society of North America meeting in Chicago when my mother called to tell me my dad had passed blood in his urine and had been diagnosed with a large left kidney cancer after receiving a CT scan. Everyone was shocked because he looked so healthy.

Dr. Bernie Siegel's *Love, Medicine and Miracles* had just been published, and my whole family began reading it. He told a story about a diagnostic dream, and I remembered my dream occurred on the only day I had spent with my dad in the previous year. Prompted by the book I recognized the similarity between the dream and real life, and it all began to make sense to me. I am named after my dad, David Lawrence Burk, Jr.

The kidney has a similar anatomic structure to the brain, with a medullary region in the center and a surrounding cortex. I must have intuitively picked up some information from him on that visit that got translated into the dream. It made me realize that medical intuition is possible. My second dream diagnostic experience came 11 years later, in North Carolina in 1998.

> I dreamt that I had lung cancer on a chest X-ray without any symptoms.

My first reaction was it might be about someone else because of my experience with my father, so I did not immediately get a radiograph taken of myself, which would have been easy enough for me to do. I decided to wait and see if the meaning would be revealed to me.

The next week, while I was attending a Jon Kabat-Zinn mindfulness meditation workshop, my integrative medicine colleague Susan Gaylord, the program director at the University of North Carolina, insisted I needed to meet a friend of hers who was also participating. She introduced him as being just like me, because he was also a radiologist. I asked him why he came to study meditation with us, as it was unusual to have even one radiologist at such a workshop, let alone two.

I don't remember what sort of professional response I thought he would give, but I wasn't prepared for the answer. He replied that he came for personal reasons and had just been diagnosed with lung cancer. A wave of recognition immediately passed through my body, as I realized my dream had been about him, not me. I shared the precognitive dream with him and wished him well on his healing journey. I went to work the next day and had a chest X-ray taken, which was completely normal, as I expected.

KAT'S INTERPRETATION

If these were my dreams. I would define the first one as a diagnostic precognitive dream for kidney cancer, and the second one as a precognitive diagnostic dream for lung cancer, and both of them as dreaming for others because it was determined through medical testing that the dreamer had neither of these diseases. The dreams were symbolic, because they involved images, rather than being literal, with words, because Dr. Larry Burk was fluent in his own dream language and understood the dreams. However, their true meanings were not completely understood until the near future, when the precognitive aspect of the dreams came true and was medically validated.

DR. BURK'S COMMENTARY

The first experience occurred only a year after starting to keep a dream diary, which was triggered by a move to Philadelphia in 1986. That was an intense period of spiritual growth, which included finding my first metaphysical bookstore, the famous Garland of Letters on South Street, one of the few independent bookstores specializing in that genre remaining in a major city. That year I also watched Shirley MacLaine's made for TV movie series *Out on a Limb*, which introduced many spiritual concepts that I had never heard of before, such as out-of-body experiences, channeling, and psychic development.

By the time the second dream experience occurred, I was deeply immersed in co-founding Duke Integrative Medicine with Marty Sullivan, a holistic cardiologist who guided our academic adventures through a series of powerful prophetic dreams. MRI technologist Ann Charles and holistic educator Pali Delevitt, who appeared in Part Three, were also contributing their amazing dreams to the process, so I'd been well prepared by these colleagues a couple of decades in advance to eventually do the Breast Cancer Dreams Project.

46

Cancer or Not Cancer?

Kathleen (Kat) O'Keefe-Kanavos
and Priscilla Willard

This story is based on material in Chapter 34 of "Surviving Cancerland:
Intuitive Aspects of Healing" by Kathleen (Kat) O'Keefe-Kanavos.

"Hi Kathy, this is Priscilla Willard." The calm voice on my answering machine belied its real level of anxiety. "I'd really like to speak with you. It's rather urgent."

The hair stood up on the back of my neck. Priscilla never called me.

I immediately returned her call.

"So, you see, I have to make a choice about surgery, even though the doctors are not sure if it is cancer. They have only seen a suspicious area on my ovary that is painful. I don't know whether to go to the doctor in Boston, who wants to perform a complete hysterectomy, or the female doctor here on the Cape, who only intends to take the one ovary with the suspicious area on it. Can you speak with my guides and see what they have to say about all this? And please ask them if the spot is cancerous," Priscilla explained calmly, while I had a panic attack on her behalf just listening to her.

"Patricia [Priscilla's cousin] and I were so impressed with how helpful and accurate the 'guides' were when her son, Tom, went through his abdominal surgeries. I hope they'll talk to you about me."

"Of course, I'll try to contact your guides," I said. "I'll call you as soon as I know something."

I covered my face with my hands. How could she explain all that so calmly? I would have been in tears. I would have been in hysterics! The C word—CANCER—still scares the hell out of me, even when it isn't my own.

That night I set my intention to dream for Priscilla. A pop-up window appeared as soon as I started to dream, and it became frozen in place, much like a TV program put on pause. My experience with previous guided dreams had taught me that this was the signal that I was entering the guided dream zone described as Dr. Einstein's Time Continuum.

Pop-up Window Dream Signal

The dream pop-up window signals to me that my dream will shift into a guided dream. The pop-up window elongates and becomes a Sacred Dream Door, through which step a number of my cloaked Franciscan monk guides, who motion for me to follow them back through the Sacred Dream Doorway. I have no idea where we are going until I step into what I call the Room Between Realms.

The room is like a celestial waiting room or conference room between the realms of the living and the dead, where the living, dead, angels, and spirit guides can gather to share information and occasionally visit. There is no time here, only space, where white floors and walls come together without borders. But in order to enter this Room Between Realms through the Sacred Doorways, you must have permission from your spirit guides, guardian angels, which they get from God. The Law of Permission rules this Dream Realm, where nothing happens or is said without an invitation and the explicit YES from the Power Above.

"Why do you want us to give you information that will be confirmed by tests?" A guide asks, hood up to conceal his face and hands folded into the long cloak sleeves. "We do not do hoops, and neither do you."

Well, that is rather direct, I think.

I explain how I feel unsure of my medical readings for others, and if I could give a reading that could be quickly validated by medical tests, it would boost my intuitive confidence. "If helping others through dreams is something I should be doing, then please help me build the confidence to be successful."

After a long pause, the single word "Okay" is uttered.

"Yes, the spot on her ovary is cancerous but contained, so it doesn't matter whether she removes just the ovary or her uterus and both ovaries, because only the one ovary is affected."

"It won't make any difference if everything else is removed or left intact. She will live the same healthy life," a different grinning guide says to me.

He is not dressed as a Franciscan monk but rather as an ancient Asian man in colorful red-and-white silk robes. He has long, white, braided hair with a matching braided beard. My dream has shifted to my marble meditation platform in the sky, and he has walked up to me on a path made of white clouds. I am pretty sure he is not one of my guides because my guides look like Franciscan monks or Druids with brown hooded robes, knotted rope belts, and sandals. I seldom see my guides' faces because they keep their hoods up. Perhaps this guide belongs to Priscilla.

"There is more," my monk guide says, leaning toward me, as if to whisper. "Priscilla will get a very bad life-threatening infection from the sutures because they were mismarked." He turns to walk away but calls over his shoulder. "Yes, all the sutures from all the operation that day must be replaced."

I awoke and reached for my dream journal to write down every single detail.

"Oh, yes, that was Ning. I have been feeling him around me," Priscilla said, when I told her what the Asian guide had said and described him. Her guide has a name; mine has a hood. Different people, different guides.

"Well, I have decided to go with the Cape doctor who only wants to take the one ovary because she doesn't think there is cancer involved, just a cyst," Priscilla said. "You will be having radiation at the time of my surgery."

"I'll put you in my radiation meditation." The words were out of my mouth before I had time to realize they may have frightened her with the thought of radiation beams and her surgery in the same meditation bubble.

"That will be wonderful. Thank you," she answered.

So, after Priscilla's ovary was sent to pathology it was found to be cancerous. She was wheeled back into surgery, and her other ovary and uterus were removed. Pathology said those had no traces of cancer. It was just as the spiritual guides had said: it didn't matter if she had a complete hysterectomy or not.

The next day Priscilla's cousin, Patricia, called me.

"Anyhow, dear, the reason I'm calling is Priscilla has popped a fever, and the doctors don't know why. They can't seem to locate an infection. Priscilla's daughter called to say Priscilla wondered if you could speak with her guide to see what is going on?"

"Sure," I told Patricia. "I think it is the sutures the guides were talking about in my dream that made no sense at the time. Tell Priscilla's daughter to ask the doctor to check the stitches he used that he thought were the dissolving kind. I don't believe they are, and they may be causing an infection and the fever. I'll call you back as soon as I know something."

"Are you sure you are up to this? I don't want you to overtire yourself." Patricia was concerned for my health, because although coming to the end of my radiation treatment brought me joy, it also brought a depth of fatigue I had never experienced before.

"No problem. I can contact her guides from my comfy bed," I answered and hung up. Priscilla's guide was waiting to speak with me.

The Asian Guide

I am halfway through my meditation when I fall into a deep sleep. Priscilla's Asian guide shows up and takes me to Priscilla's hospital room, where I meet many people who are "in spirit" (dead) and watching over Priscilla. They greet me, introducing themselves by name as soon as I astral-traveled in, all speaking at once, then stand together, as if posing for pictures and say, "Tell her we're in the album."

After I left Priscilla's room in the dream, I called Patricia and told her about "the visitors."

"I just finished speaking with Priscilla's daughter, and she doesn't know who the people are you saw in Priscilla's hospital room," Patricia said over the telephone, "but it turns out that you are right, the infection *is* in the stitches, and they did use the wrong type of sutures. Apparently, they were mislabeled or something, and the doctor must remove them from a number of patients. It is unbelievable what goes on in a hospital, but even more unbelievable is how the guides got that information.

"But tell me about the people in the hospital room, because Priscilla said the nurse you described with the short, curly, black hair is her nurse. So you were in the right place. You told me you saw the living nurse in black and white while the 'passed-over spirits' in the room were in color?"

Black-and-White Spirits

I explain how midway through my meditation I fell asleep and found myself in Priscilla's hospital room, rather than my special place in the sky. Priscilla was asleep, while the room was full of people dressed in colorful clothing conversing with one another. However, the nurse was in black and white and seemed oblivious to the commotion in the room.

"I practically astral-traveled on top of the nurse when I entered the room."

"Hi. Priscilla has a bad infection in her sutures because they are the wrong kind. They don't dissolve. It's going to take her six months to recover from this complication. She needs a new doctor, too. I don't like the one she has," an attractive lady in her 30s with shiny shoulder-length brown hair and dressed in 1950s clothing said to me once I reclaimed my composure.

"What do you think, dear?" she asked, turning to a handsome gentleman peering down at Penny.

"Yes, I quite agree. But we will stay until she is better, which should be soon."

"Who are you?" I finally managed to ask, surprised by the people, their conversation, and their automatic assumption that I had expected to see them and knew who they were. And they seemed to know me.

"Oh, we're family. I'm Linda. This is my husband, Kevin," she said of the tall, dark-haired gentleman who turned and smiled at the mention of his name. "And our son, Jeff," she said, a boy who appeared to be about 17 years of age, tall with dark hair. He was standing beside his mother and had not spoken a word the whole time.

At this point, they all moved closer together, with their son in the middle, and struck a pose. "We're in the family album," she said with a smile, just before my guide showed up and whisked me back home to my body and bed.

In the following days, the infection from the sutures affected Priscilla's heart, and she was admitted to the intensive care unit. Somehow (I'm sure it was with the help of our guides), Patricia and I snuck in to see her and told her what the guides had said about a six-month recovery. I held her hand while Patricia stood at the foot of the bed and cupped Priscilla's feet in her hands.

"If you are not family you cannot be in here!" The nurse said, surprised we had slipped past her.

"Oh, we're family," Patricia white-lied. Or did she? And we left, confident that Priscilla knew she would live.

And she did. Six months later, she was back to her old self. But before she was released from the hospital, her daughter called to tell me Priscilla had told her where to find the family album. It contained the deceased family members who had visited her in the hospital, with the date and their names beautifully written on the back. In the old black-and-white photo, they were posed in the exact same position described in the dream.

KAT'S INTERPRETATION

The dream is precognitive, because it foretells of infected sutures; diagnostic, because of its diagnosis of cancer; and healing, because it gives healing advice to survive infection and cancer. Although this dream is literal, because it is filled with direct conversation for guidance by spiritual guides, it does still contain symbolism, as if for additional validation. A *window* in a dream may symbolize insight (a play on words) or your outlook or perspective on some aspect of life. You look in and out of a window. *Doors* may symbolize a transition from one stage or situation in life to another. In this dream, the window was an insight to a transitional place, which provided a positive outlook on a challenging life.

Priscilla's spirit guide, Ning, has braided hair on his head and face and is dressed in flowing red-and-white robes.

Hair represents thoughts that come from the head. Hair on the face can be a play on words—thoughts at face value. Long hair symbolizes divinity. Hair in braids represents neat and orderly thought, determination, and a strong mindset. *Silver or white hair* represents the purity of thought. The color white and red represents pure power while flowing robes is a symbol of joyful celebration. Ning represents orderly, divine thought at face value, wrapped in powerful joy.

A black-and-white dream has significant dual meaning. *Black* may signify a mystery, the unconscious, mourning, and potential. The color *white* in dreams may mean the conscious mind, purity, rebirth, and potential.

I am often asked, "Why is the live nurse in the hospital room seen in black and white, while the dead visitors were seen in color." There are multiple explanations for this phenomenon. One answer is that we converse with the dead in their realm. The living seen through the eyes of the dead can be viewed as an old black-and-white movie. When the dead family members were found in the album, they were black and white. It could be validation. Another explanation may be that I was seeing Priscilla through the eyes of the dreaming dead family.

Dream research suggests the type of television you watched as a child has a profound effect on the color of your dreams.[65] Research from 1915 through to the 1950s showed that while almost all people under the age of 25 dream in color, thousands over the age of 55, who were brought up with black-and-white TV sets, often dream in monochrome, even now. Those born before TV existed looked at black-and white-photos. Eva Murzyn, a psychology student at Dundee University, UK, was one of the researchers who carried out this study on technicolor vs. monochrome dreams. The family in Priscilla's hospital room lived in the 1940s. Perhaps I was seeing them through their eyes.

DR. BURK'S COMMENTARY

Kat's ability to set an intention to get health information in a dream and then have the dreamworld actually deliver it is quite a remarkable skill, especially when the information comes from an unfamiliar guide and deceased relatives. It is really a form of medical intuition, a topic I have been researching for the past 25 years.[66] Medical intuitives like Caroline Myss and my teaching partner at the Monroe Institute, Winter Robinson, are able to access diagnostic information while in the waking state. Others, like Edgar Cayce, could only make diagnoses in a trance state. It is a natural talent that can be developed with practice. However, much more research is required for it to gain acceptance in conventional medicine.

47

My Son's Tethered Cord and Epilepsy Treatment

Suzanne M. De Gregorio

A theme running through the experiences of my peers in Dr. Burk's Breast Cancer Dreams Project is slowing down during and after treatment, going deep within the self for guidance and answers. For me, it was the opposite. My world sped up. You see, I wasn't just fighting for my own life; I had to save my son.

Alex has epilepsy and other neurological problems that cause immense pain. He woke up screaming, went to bed screaming, and screamed most of the hours between. He unraveled for years. I could not work because when Alex attacked other children, which was often, I had to get him from school. This child was out of his mind with pain but unable to tell us what hurt.

Overwhelmed by lights and sounds, my son could not stand to be in public, effectively rendering us housebound. When we did go out, and the neurological firestorms activated, needing something to grab onto, he'd occasionally pull me into the back seat of the car by my hair while I was driving. Alex bit his arms up and down until they bruised.

I began dreaming.

Alex's Accident

Alex was in horrific accidents, then got up and walked away as if nothing happened. Once he drove a truck off a cliff and emerged without a scratch. Another time, I watched in horror as he fell from a several-story balcony onto concrete. He lay motionless and contorted for a bit, then stood up and walked off.

After this, I began paying closer attention to the quality of my predictive dreams, looking for patterns and connecting dots. This work was an asset when a waking dream concerning Alex seized my life. Foreshadowing dreams, for me, are those that recur, so I knew we had a bumpy ride ahead.

Alex began having trouble walking. My son always had gastrointestinal problems, so a lumbar MRI was ordered, along with magnetic imaging of the hip. A benign tumor was found on his hip, but Alex's spinal cord was tethered. Our cords lie gently within our spinal columns but are never meant to stretch. Bound up since the womb, poor Alex's cord was pulling as he grew, causing immense pain. After corrective surgery, he got up and walked, just as he had in my dreams.

A postmortem of life imitating these dreams taught me a key lesson. Bereft that something horrible was about to befall my baby, I neglected imagery from both dreams of Alex getting up and walking away unscathed. Offering this hopeful aspect space in my distressed psyche could have neutralized excessive worry early on. I have since learned to count all potentially precognitive dream data as relevant.

My son's health issues are like peeling an onion: one problem squared away, only to reveal another layer beneath. His epilepsy medication, though helpful, was never enough to stabilize his brain. One day, I threw myself on the ground sobbing, begging for answers.

Words are inadequate to describe what happened next. Time seemed distorted, and my mind silenced. I felt the following information imprint wordlessly within me.

Around the time of puberty, something will come along that will be a game changer for Alex, but you must pay close attention, or you will miss it.

Alex was 10 years old. This was new. I was accustomed to working with dream-derived prophetic information, but this incident suggested I'd have to search for my answers in waking reality.

Excited by the healing prospects for Alex, each day I scanned for clues, medical abstracts, and news articles in a needle-in-a-haystack attempt to find his miracle, when I stumbled upon Dr. Sanjay Gupta's CNN documentary, *Weed*. I saw an astonishing improvement of pediatric epilepsy from the cannabis plant. Alex was now 11, nearing puberty.

We live in Louisville, Kentucky, not California or Colorado, and the plant was illegal here. Why should my son be deprived of his best chance because we lived in the wrong zip code? I started investigating the legislative process, learning what needed to be done to gain access to the hemp oil.

Alex Speaks

Around that time, I dreamed Alex was talking to me in fluent sentences. That week, my sister called, telling me she dreamed that Alex was talking with her. And my friend Kathryn dreamed that she walked next to my son as he rode a bike. He told her how hard it was when he had autism.

One week. Three people. Similar dreams. This oil was it! This would be Alex's game changer. Something had to be done. I pulled together a team of parents of children with epilepsy and got the state's epilepsy advocacy group on board. We got the law. Within four months cannabinoid oil, or CBD, was technically legal in Kentucky. However, discrepancies between state and federal law still deprived children of their medicine. So my focus shifted to helping change federal medical cannabis law, which has yet to pass.

My chemo injection station became a mobile command center for my part in a national grassroots parent effort to federally legalize medical cannabis. A researcher once sat all day with me during an infusion. We bounced ideas off each other. I would often be on the phone with Senator Paul's, Senator McConnell's, and Congressman Yarmuth's offices as oncology nurses injected Taxotere, Carboplatin, and Herceptin into my system. When I hung up, my fellow patients were full of questions. Do you think you can win? You'd be amazed how popular a topic medical cannabis is in the chemo ward.

My son eventually got his game changer, right on time, at 13 years of age, just as he entered puberty. It has been a miracle. After starting CBD with his neurologist's approval, Alex had the first clear EEG in his life. Gone are the day-long tantrums, the aggression, constant headaches, and he talks more now. My son started riding a bike within three weeks of taking the oil, just as in Kathryn's dream. And he talks to us. Boy, does he talk!

One day, as the time for his dose drew near, my son said, "I need my oil for my brain."

> **KAT'S INTERPRETATION**
>
> Suzanne was fantastic at understanding her precognitive dreams about her son, which were validated by medical tests.

DR. BURK'S COMMENTARY

I was a co-author on one of the earliest papers on the use of MRI for the diagnosis of tethered spinal cord in children. which is sometimes apparent due to the presence of other congenital spinal deformities, but other times can be delayed until later in life due to difficulty walking, as in Alex's case. Suzanne's dream of his eventual healing through surgery certainly set the stage for her experience with his epilepsy.

The use of cannabinoid oil in the treatment of intractable childhood seizure disorders has been a major breakthrough in recent years and a major impetus for the legalization of medical marijuana products around the country. Her initial precognitive guidance came in the form of a waking dream, which was reinforced by the dream of him speaking once she started down the path to legislative activism. It was amazing that his healing process intersected with hers during chemotherapy in a very synchronistic way. Some things are meant to be, and dreams remind us of how mysterious healing can happen.

48

Deadly Heart Attack

Jane Katra, PhD

This story involves three extraordinarily gifted individuals: health educator and spiritual healer Jane Katra; Russell Targ, laser physicist and remote viewing expert; and his deceased daughter, Elizabeth, who prior to her untimely death from a brain tumor was a leading integrative medicine physician doing research on the health benefits of prayer.

February 2017

Hi Russell,

I had a compelling dream visit with you in the astral early this morning. In the dream, Elizabeth showed me a shocking image of you, conveying to me that you were not 100 percent well. She emphasized to me that your condition was something that I could see, but that you weren't paying attention to at all. She stressed that you could not feel that you had a problem.

The words that came to me were, "It's like a silent problem." That's why I'm sending you this email. In any case, I was shocked at your appearance that she showed me.

Then I Was with You in the Dream

I told you your appearance was not right at all. I was seeing your torso all bloated up, with brown and green splotchy skin. (My thoughts were: *Green, gangrene, tissues being starved of oxygen.*) My thought, in the dream, was maybe your heart is not pumping strongly enough.

Then I leaned over and put my heart up close to yours, and a huge whoosh of energy burst out, and I was jolted awake.

I knew I was meant to contact you and tell you about this... I hope you are well. Do take care.

Blessings and Love,
Jane

Russell Targ emailed me back, saying he was feeling just fine, which is exactly how Elizabeth had told me he would react. (Elizabeth is Russell's deceased daughter in spirit, who had been an MD, and who had told me on her deathbed that she was not done being a healer.)

Five days later, Russell's heart rate dropped dramatically. He reported that he "had no pain, but lots of sudden sweating, weakness, and heaviness in his chest. You'll know what that means if you experience it."

He called 911, and five paramedics in rubber boots and tons of hardware arrived at his door within five minutes. Within another minute they determined his heart rate was "near nil."

"They ripped off my tee-shirt and started shocking me with paddles in my dining room. Within eight minutes of calling 911, I was on my way to Stanford Hospital. They told me I wouldn't live long enough to get to my doctor at Kaiser. The paramedics called ahead to Stanford, and they were waiting for us when we arrived at emergency."

Russell reports that he became unconscious and "had 90 minutes of extremely unpleasant electrical shocks administered to his heart," which each time brought him back to temporary consciousness. The next he remembered was being "in recovery, with a pacemaker installed, and a heart rate of 60."

Russell is now back home and feeling much better.

KAT'S INTERPRETATION

If this were my dream, I would call it a precognitive diagnostic dream where the dreamer is dreaming for others. It was precognitive, because the diagnosis was for a medical condition that would happen in the near future. It was Literal, because there was a conversation within the dream, with symbolism in the form of a play on words, "It's like a silent problem." And "tissues being starved of oxygen," which happens during a heart attack. The dream diagnosis was for someone other than the dreamer, yet confirmed by a medical report.

DR. BURK'S COMMENTARY

I was present many years ago when Jane was first contacted by Elizabeth through Mary Jo Bulbrook, an intuitive nurse healer who also is a medium. Deceased relatives who appear in dreams bearing valuable medical information were a common occurrence in the breast cancer support group interviewed by Wanda Burch in 2004.

49

The X-rays

Kathi Kemper, MD, MPH

Lately, I've been inspired to get really into dreams, faithfully recording the dreams and my initial interpretation daily.

> Yesterday, part of one of the dreams involved a dear friend and colleague, TL, who I dreamed I helped get the kidney she needed for her transplant, as her kidneys were failing. (I have no conscious knowledge that she has kidney problems, but like you, Kat, she is a three-time cancer survivor, ovarian in her case.)
>
> In the dream, I saw her in the hospital surrounded by her daughter, grandmother (who was translucent, so I assumed she had passed), and other friends, happy and loved. Then I saw her X-rays and knew she had a right hip replacement due to martial arts injuries when younger (again no conscious knowledge of that). But when I looked at the X-ray, it was fine, normal, no arthritis at all.

When I awoke, I realized, of course, that the dream could be all about me but decided to send that part to her just in case. She wrote back immediately and confirmed her kidneys are declining in function due to chemo side effects, but she's not in failure yet; her grandmother had passed, but she felt her loving presence very strongly; and her right hip had been replaced due to martial arts injuries but is fine now. She found the dream very reassuring and helped her feel peaceful, since I saw things coming together for her and how she was surrounded by so much love. How about that?

KAT'S INTERPRETATION

If this were my dream, I might think it were a symbolic diagnostic dream about me also, but Kathi decided to take a chance and share the dream with the person she suspected it was for and was rewarded with an affirmative reply. Dr. Kathi Kemper was dreaming for another. The dream was actually literal, because it showed Kathi X-rays and other literal medical information about the patient, which was also validation.

DR. BURK'S COMMENTARY

It is interesting that she had no conscious knowledge of the hip prosthesis or the compromised kidney function that was detected in the dream. Sometimes, the Dreamworld just gives you exactly what you need at the time. The translucent deceased grandmother reminds me of the final celebration scene in the original *Star Wars* trilogy, where Yoda, Obi-Wan Kenobi, and Anakin Skywalker all appear as ghostly figures. I wonder what kind of dreams about the Force guided George Lucas in producing that epic saga?

50

Ovarian Cancer –
Mary's Client's Story

It was probably five years ago when my client, a retired physician, came to see me for an intuitive consultation. I too practice medical intuition. While scanning her body, her lower abdomen "felt off" to me, much like my breast in the previous story (Chapter 15) had felt off to me. In other words, the energy felt dark in her abdomen. When asked if she had had an internal exam recently, she answered no. She would, however, have her belly looked at.

That night I had a dream.

Cancer Looks Like Hair

I was just falling asleep, in that twilight area between fully awake and completely asleep, when the memory of my client's session came into my dream, along with a book I had read, *Hands of Light* by Barbara Brennan. The book was open to the page that shows how cancer looks like hair, and as I dropped into a deeper sleep, it made me wonder if this was a message telling me my client had cancer.

A couple of years went by before she called and said she should have listened to me and gone to the doctor earlier. My client was diagnosed with ovarian cancer. She asked me not to contact her; she would reach out when she was ready.

Last year, while having morning coffee, she came to mind. It was almost as if she were in the room with me. It felt peaceful. I thought, *I will email her*, although I also thought, *Oh, God. Maybe she is no longer here*. Ten minutes after sending her an email, I got a response from her sister, saying my client had passed away a couple months prior. Life is sure interesting, as are dreams.

KAT'S INTERPRETATION

If this were my dream, I would define it as a symbolic diagnostic precognitive dream for someone else, because Mary's dream is about her client. Mary is the dream messenger. The validation for the dream was the client's death from cancer.

DR. BURK'S COMMENTARY

Mary's experience is an example of a medical intuitive process begun in the waking state continuing to its diagnostic conclusion in the dream state. If her client had taken action on the initial intuitive impression, she might have been able to catch the cancer at a more treatable stage, since early detection is critical with ovarian tumors, as in the previous example shared by Kat. It is also worth mentioning that Barbara Brennan has trained many healers throughout the world in developing their medical intuition. Her books, full of dramatic visual imagery, have inspired others to work on their clairvoyant skills.

PART NINE

*Conclusion and Vision for
the Future, with Prevention, Intuitive
Guidance, and Spiritual Implications*

Nobody doubts the importance of conscious experience;
why then should we doubt the significance of unconscious happenings?
They also are part of our life, and sometimes more truly a part of it
for weal or woe than any happenings of the day.
— **CARL JUNG,** *CW 16, Para 325*

51

"Your Cables Are Twisted"

Kathleen (Kat) O'Keefe-Kanavos

> *The patient, that is to say, does not need to have a truth*
> *inculcated into him—if we do that, we only reach his head; he needs*
> *far more to grow up to this truth, and in that way we reach his heart,*
> *and the appeal goes deeper and works more powerfully.*
> — CARL JUNG, *CW 16m Para 314*

All the diagnostic and precognitive dreams in this book either saved lives, or had the potential to save them, if the dreams were taken seriously. Imagine if many of the dreamers, myself included, did not have to self-advocate to the point of being obnoxious, or wait months for tests they knew they needed from the information in their dreams. Consider, if you will, using dreams to find an illness in its earliest stage, to increase your chances of survival, and allow your treatments to be less radical.

It took three months to get the exploratory surgery I needed the first time to find stage 2 aggressive breast cancer, which was in one lymph node. This resulted in two more surgeries, chemotherapy, and radiation; the loss of all my hair; and taking Tamoxifen for five years, which stopped working after two years. But that is another dream story for the next book.

Now, imagine if I had felt secure enough to tell my doctor, "I had a dream..." and had an MRI three months earlier that discovered cancer at a much earlier stage. My treatment may have been less invasive, painful, and produced fewer side effects. I believe when we bombard our body with toxins to give ourselves more time on this end of our lifeline, we take time off the other end. Chemotherapy is not a healthy walk in the park. It is deadly last measure treatment to save a life.

Dreams can make the difference between early and late detection of any disease, which can make the difference between life and death, as validated by the stories of illnesses in this book. Most were described as asymptomatic and diagnostic dreams were the only symptoms and warning signs that something was wrong.

It has been 18 years since my first dreams of cancer, and almost 15 since my second and third cancers, all of which were asymptomatic except for my dreams. This has given me a stronger sense of confidence concerning my ability to use dreams as a diagnostic tool.

The following recounts why and how I now tell my diagnostic dreams to the healing community.

After a recent coast-to-coast flight in a chilly jet, for the first time ever I developed excruciating pain in my right buttock, which radiated down my leg, creating severe thigh and calf cramps and numbness in my right foot. Unable to sit or bend my body, I went to the emergency room, where I was diagnosed with Piriformis Syndrome, which is a lesion of the sciatic nerve. Given the choice of an anesthetic/corticosteroid injection in my sore butt or a prescription for a muscle relaxant, I chose the pills. I do not like needles! The doctor told me it would take six months for the condition to entirely correct itself.

That night I had a dream.

"Your Cables Are Twisted"

There is a big beach party, and I am in charge of filming the festivities live from a giant two-story TV camera stationed down on the beach, where it sends the picture by way of large electrical cables up a steady, sloping, grassy hill to another gigantic TV set at the top of the hill, perched high on a platform, where it is monitored. The picture on the uphill TV has pixels missing and blank spots that are shorting out.

As I try to figure out what is wrong, using the dials, a man calls up to me and says, "Your cables are twisted and tangled. They are folding back on themselves and shorting out the wires and cords inside. You need to pull them straight and have them running parallel down the hill to connect the pictures."

I descend the stairs of the platform to the grass and stand on three of the 12 tangled cords.

"You have to take your shoes off, or you'll make them worse," he says.

I look down to see I'm wearing my white Chanel sandals with wooden heels. I kick them off and begin the back-breaking process of picking up the heavy, 1-foot-diameter cords, untangling them by pulling them straight and laying them back down parallel to each other. As I look down the hill, I realize this is going to be a long hard job.

The next morning my pain is still so profound, I make an appointment for a massage. Rosemary, the therapist, greets me with, "How can I help you?"

I surprise myself when I answer with, "I had a dream last night," rather than offering her the medical diagnosis.

"Wonderful! Tell me your dream."

I left out no dream details, and Rosemary said, "I know just what is wrong by your dream. You have an injured piriformis, which is playing havoc with your sciatic nerve. Are you experiencing cramps in your calf and numbness in your foot?"

She then pointed to a picture of the human muscular system hanging on the wall and asked me to show her where the pain was in my buttocks. It was labeled *The Piriformis*.[67, 68, 69]

Rosemary then pointed to the "muscle cords" running down the leg like cables on the chart, which in my dream were running down the hill. She then proceeded to massage my cords, so they relaxed and straightened themselves out releasing the pain and neuropathy in my foot. I recovered in six weeks rather than six months and was back on the tennis court, and I never took the muscle relaxants, because they made me nauseous.

The earlier an illness or condition is diagnosed, the better the chances for full recovery. This book proves dreams are an amazing diagnostic and healing tool. How wonderful would it be to walk into a convention medical office and say to the doctor, "I had a dream" and have the physician smile and say, "Tell me your dream," and use it as a diagnostic tool for further testing and treatment as a direct or indirect result of Dr. Larry Burk's Research Groups?

It is our hope that this book is a giant step in making that dream come true.

52

"The Hero's Journey into the Underworld"

Larry Burk, MD, CEHP

Any classic story of adventure in movies, novels, or epic folktales follows the model of the hero's journey described by mythologist Joseph Campbell.[70] There are many steps in his monomyth model, including life in the ordinary world; the call to adventure; refusal of the call; discovering a mentor; passing the threshold; finding allies and encountering enemies, tests, and challenges; approaching the innermost cave; seizing the sword; the ultimate ordeal; resurrection; and returning with the elixir.

When I left my academic position at Duke in 2004 to do teleradiology from home and pursue my adventures in healing on my own, I never thought I would return. However, in early October 2015, I got an unexpected invitation to come back to my old musculoskeletal imaging section to work part-time, as my former colleagues were very short-staffed and had more work reading X-rays than they knew what to do with. The night of October 5, I wrote this question in my dream diary, "Should I work at Duke part-time?"

> I dream that I arrive at a classroom on a college campus. A woman teacher appears, who reminds me of my favorite English teacher from my Duke undergrad days in the 1970s. She says this will be an exciting adventure in creative writing! I didn't know I had signed up for that.
>
> I start off on a hero's journey down a winding road and encounter a mysterious old woman at a roadside stand. She sells me a glass drink bottle. I start to drink the magic elixir and notice writing on the inside of the label revealed through the dark liquid.
>
> I follow the instructions there to go into an elevator and push the down button. It descends into the underworld, and I get out at the lowest level. I step out into a new adventure and hear the words, "We are off to see the wizard!"

I accepted the offer to return to Duke with a starting date in December. During my orientation week, I had the precognitive bike accident dream experience described in Chapter 32, with the theme of resilience. The healing elixir I drank while being guided to resurrect my Duke career has given me the ability to do further research on breast cancer dreams in a more formal academic setting. Now that the writing of this book is complete, I can pick up my intellectual sword again and start the next pilot project on dreams of women who are having breast biopsies.

As you read the many amazing stories in the book, you probably recognized the theme of the hero's journey in many of them. Hopefully, you will be better equipped with your dream diary, guides, and perhaps even a magic feather to embark on your own hero's journey. Or maybe you are already in the middle of one and are undergoing the ultimate ordeal. May you find your sword and healing elixir during the process of resurrection!

53

If I Knew Then What I Know Now –
Words of Wisdom and
Encouragement for You

One looks back with appreciation to the brilliant teachers,
but with gratitude to those who touched our human feelings.
The curriculum is so much necessary raw material,
but warmth is the vital element for the growing plant
and for the soul of the child.

— CARL JUNG

The premise for this chapter is you. After sharing how we dreamed our way to wellness in Dr. Larry Burk's Breast Cancer Dreams Project, it is our pleasure to share our Words of Wisdom and encouragement with you. If we only knew then what we know now, what would we want to share with the world to make the journey we were destined to travel a little bit easier, successful, and fulfilling for you? Some of us thought long and hard about sharing our wisdom; others immediately knew what to say. These little Pearls of Wisdom are also keys to dreams, health, and healing success.

Pearls of Wisdom?

A thread ran through many cancer dream stories in the book. It was the symbolism of crabs, spiders, calcifications, and other irritants in the lives of the dreamers, such as "Three Crabs, Three Pearls, and a Physician-within" by Kathleen (Kat) O'Keefe-Kanavos.

What are pearls except for the beautiful transformation of life's irritants into layers of treasure? Pearls begin as grains of sand, similar to calcifications in the breast, or foreign toxic invaders like tiny baby crabs, inserting themselves into the soft tissues of a mollusk with the intention of eating the oyster alive, from the inside out. In response to the potentially life-threatening situations, the mollusk contains the irritant by encapsulating it.

Over time, it is transformed into a beautiful, highly prized gem called a natural pearl—the tangible positive outcome of an adverse situation. Pearls are worn as men's tie-pins and the treasured Jackie Kennedy full necklace. If a pearl could speak, what layers of stories would it share? In the Words of Wisdom below, we gift our Pearls of Wisdom to you. Wear your pearls with pride.

"Go to the Depths of Your Being."
— **CAROLYN K KINNEY**, *PhD, RN*

Sharing what I have gained with you enables me to more fully integrate my experiences, to interweave the fabric of my body, mind, and spirit, and to continue with the never-ending process of reconstructing my self. Sometimes, in struggling to understand it all, it is helpful to go to the depths of your being to examine the whys and hows of what is happening. Death and severe illness of self or a loved one often brings one's life and purpose more fully into examination and question. Death and grief cause us to speculate about our own mortality, and we are reminded that nothing is permanent in this world, the visible world.

Reevaluate what is important and what you hope to accomplish, not just in your professional career but in your life. Slowly begin to make substantial changes in the way you approach life; specifically, start to pay more attention to your own needs, as well as the needs of others you love. You may experience many losses associated with the significant changes that may occur from your changes. Know that grieving and losses are necessary if you are going to be able to move forward in a healthy way. Allow yourself time for this to happen.

I asked myself over and over, "How can I look at what has happened in a way that is healthy and growth-directed?" The answer came as I heard my inner voice repeating the opening paragraph of Charles Dickens's *A Tale of Two Cities:*

It was the best of times, it was the worst of times, it was the age of wisdom, It was the age of foolishness, it was the epoch of belief, it was the epoch of incredulity, it was the season of Light, it was the season of Darkness, it was the spring of hope, it was the winter of despair.

Perhaps the most important component of a new course of life is addressing your spiritual needs.

"I Am Alive Because of My Dreams."
— WANDA BURCH

What I learned, and wished I had known then (but pleased that I know now), is that dreaming is a continuing dialogue with the inner self, a constantly streaming two-way message center, the inner voice, and inner-physician, that speaks to us in sleep, dreams, or through the imagination; the voice that knows us best and allows us access once we relax and allow the day's intrusions to peel away.

Any creative use of the imagination has the potential for participation in the healing process. Whether we are awake or asleep, imagery, or mind pictures, is the way we send messages to our body, releasing the most creative and powerful potential of our subconscious, providing an intention for healing that empowers the imagination to transport healing messages to the body.

Personal imagery taps our own experience but explores far beyond our waking experience, making all things possible inside and outside the boundaries of time and space. It is there that we can sort and choose the messages that will contribute most powerfully to our healing. Actively drawing upon those images, we can write a story, create a meditation for ourselves or others, sing a song, explore personal myth, dance, draw, manipulate a creative form on a computer, form an image out of clay, reenter a dream, or take an image from a dream. The totality of the experience—story within dreaming, art, music, exercise, a walk in nature—brings healing to the body, the mind, and the spirit.

In order to fully heal, we must engage all the places within the heart, soul, mind, and body that are inspired by the imagination, so that doors for healing are opened. We need to look for our life dreams—the ones that can be actively expressed in all forms of creativity and in every part of the imagination. Using imaginal resources in conjunction with traditional medicine and with traditional complementary therapies vastly expands the boundaries of our personal healing process. Using the imagination in healing is within reach of every human being on Earth.

"Be Brave When Confronting Intuitive Dreams."
— SUZANNE DE GREGORIO

It is tempting to ignore the warnings of intuitive dreams because we would rather not believe ourselves or someone we love is at risk. The consequence of that might be dire. Pay attention also to other aspects of the dream, not just the scary, dramatic stuff. Nestled in there too can be suggestions that things will ultimately be alright. Focusing on those issues could reassure you, as the little whale did for Diane and the promise to Sunni that she'd reenter the race where she left off. And the journey need not end with hints that come unbidden in the night. My cancer warning dreams were but an opening wedge to greater healing possibilities. I'm now taking it a step further: learning to dialogue with my sleeping self to heal my body.

Tests found autonomic nervous system dysregulation, likely from chemotherapy.

> As symptoms set in, I dreamed my garage was leveled in a tornado. It was
> reconstructed but without a foundation.

For me, dreams of houses have always related to my body, with garages representing my brain. The symbolism was clear: unless I built a strong foundation, though I may look fine outwardly, my neurological health would be precarious.

Research implied paleo diet, intermittent fasting, and increasing exercise could help regenerate autonomic nerves by improving mitochondrial function. I committed religiously to this lifestyle for a year.

> About eight months in, drifting off to sleep, I found myself in a garage far
> more attractive than my own, with scrubbed white walls and sunlit windows.
> I dropped to the floor and began spreading the foundation.

With Wanda Burch's book, *She Who Dreams,* as my guide, I worked with this imagery every day, visualizing myself in that attractive garage, spreading the foundation. A year after the detection of my autonomic nervous system dysfunction, I went to Vanderbilt University for more in-depth testing. The neurologist there found my autonomic nervous function grossly intact.

It is to the point now where I can sometimes hold a question before bed and receive a visual image in response as I drift off to sleep or during a dream. It is symbolism that I must decode, so this phenomenon still makes me work; it is ever evolving, expecting more of me before I get to access the next level. This is not some superpower, but the product dedicated to focusing across time.

Tell everyone, including people at a hospital who will listen, if you have had a medical dream diagnosing an illness, because I am still reeling from the fact that such a thing can happen. Accept that comprehensive self-care is everything. Not just in one area of your life but across the board—mind, body, and spirit. Meditate every day, and be pretty inflexible about that. Yoga has changed my life. Sometimes—actually most of the time for me—a dream is just a dream. So learning to decipher the precognitive dream from other dreams that are just processing fear has been a challenge. Still, it is work worth doing.

"Spend More Time Connecting to Self."
— SUNNI INGALLS

If I had known then what I know now, I would have found the time for "me" long ago. Each moment, I would have lived more fully, more present, nourishing my body and soul. I would have really heard what others were saying and not have been so wrapped up in what my response was going to be. I would have been more open to new experiences and less fearful of the unknown.

Yoga would have been a daily practice to balance my mind, body, and spirit and not just a stretch. The "noise" of my children would have been heard as music, cleaning would have been a dance, and cooking a moving meditation.

I would have also forgiven myself for the moments that I was unable to live with that level of gratitude and presence. I would have forgiven myself for *all* the "mistakes" I had made in my life, and recognized the gift of wisdom that each experience provided me.

More time would have been spent connecting to myself, my family, friends, strangers, nature, and all that is life (God for me). I believe that healing comes from all of these things: presence, balance, gratitude, forgiveness, and connection. And when we can incorporate these attributes into our daily life, we find fulfillment and peace. Eventually, every cell in our body recognizes this harmony, and it is then that we are in a perfect state of health.

Listen to your intuition and pay attention to your dreams. Don't dismiss dreams or feelings that are strong or "stick with you." That is how I describe my "prophetic/message" dreams. Take time to just sit with the thought or dream. Don't attach to it, but ask yourself some questions, like if you should act on it, follow up with a doctor, and so forth, then honor yourself by following through with what you come up with.

"Doctors and Specialists Make Mistakes."
— SONIA LEE-SHIELD

If there's one thing I could impart to everyone it is that doctors and specialists make mistakes, and when your inner voice starts screaming or dreaming you should listen.

"Dreams Can Solve Problems."
— AMPARO TRUJILLO AND ROCIO AGUIRRE

Delving further into our dreams allows us to find out, reveal, or uncover those hidden messages from the unconscious mind to benefit from them. By exploring our dreams, we can tap into our deepest desires, talents, and skills, as well as our fears and limiting beliefs. They can guide us to solve problems and warn us about physical illness.

Dreams speak in the language of images, symbols, and metaphors. They may seem weird or illogical, because they don't follow the linear thinking we use in the waking state, but diminishing them as irrelevant is to forget an important human treasure.

"Fight Like Hell!"
— PAULETTE WYSSBROD-GOLTZ

Acceptance of things we can't change does not mean we should not fight like hell for what we do know. What if I had acquiesced when the first doctor at the medical office only wanted to do a mammogram, the same office that failed to follow up on previous mammograms that showed calcifications, despite my substantial family history of breast cancer? If I hadn't pushed for a biopsy against their judgment, my cancer would have been caught at a later stage, and I might not be here to write this. Doctors know a lot, but they don't know everything.

Online you have at your fingertips many of the studies physicians do, but you need their help interpreting them. Read. Research. Ask questions. For instance, since my paternal grandfather, mother and two sisters had breast cancer, why did no one ever suggest an occasional MRI since mammography can miss tumors in some women? If you think you have a problem with a doctor, get a new one; it could save your life. And if you have a dream that warns you about a health condition, push it until someone listens to you, regardless of their response.

"Be a Force of Nature."
— DIANE LONG

Believe in your dreams. Be so grateful that you are breathing. Seek out new experience, live life, and be with people who make you laugh. And when you are not listened to, dare to be a force of nature.

"Dreams Are Our Allies."

— DENISE

Our dreams are an amazingly rich resource for us. We are so unbalanced in the world, and dreams are one of the ways we get the balance we need. We often think that something is important if it comes from the left side of our brain, the logical side, when the right side of our brain is where gifts like dreams reside. Pay attention to what your dreams might be trying to tell you. Keep a dream journal, and read books on dreams that go beyond dream dictionaries because it is important to learn your own dream language. All dreams come in the service of health and wholeness. Dreams are our allies. Your dreams are nightly gifts.

"Our Higher Power Speaks through Dreams."

— KATHLEEN (KAT) O'KEEFE-KANAVOS

Cancer, even recurrence, is no longer a death sentence. Often, fear of the unknown from being uninformed concerning treatment can be the real killer. If you are going through cancer treatment, the people in this book are here to tell you, "Against all the odds we did it, and you can too." Like all the amazing women and men in this book have said, "Believe in your dreams and be guided by them." To their wisdom, I would like to add: Trust in your dreams, and trust in your Higher Power, because your Higher Power often speaks to you through dreams.

Don't tell your Higher Power how big your problems are. Tell your problems how big your Higher Power is, and stand in that power.

Like Diane Long said, self-advocate, use the internet to research information and answers. Become an e-patient. *Don't* take no for an answer. *Don't* be dismissed. *Do* be a squeaky wheel until you are heard.

Just as Suzanne and Sunni shared, I believe self-care is a key to good health. Many of us are the caregivers in our families. Illness in the breast may be interpreted as a disease centered around the caregiver within. Like the airlines say, "Put your oxygen mask on first, then tend to your family and friends." You are number one! Whenever you doubt your self-worth, repeat that phrase to yourself until you feel it in your heart. As Denise said, choose to live your life with the people who make you happy. Be one of the people who make you happy.

And, to echo what Sonia Lee-Shield said, "Doctors and technicians make mistakes." But we have a Divine Default System called dreams, in which our Physician-within can guide us.

Your dreams are an innate gift from God. We are all born with spirit guides and guardian angels. We are their job, and they take that job very seriously and speak to us in dreams. I agree with Sunni, "Listen to your intuition, and pay attention to your dreams," because they can come true and save your life. The stories from these amazing women who dared to believe in their dreams are proof positive. As Carolyn K. Kinney suggested, learn from them.

Rocio Aguirre of the mother-daughter dream team shared an important fact proved by our dreams, "Delving further into our dreams allows us to find out, reveal, or uncover those hidden messages from the unconscious mind." Those messages can be lifesavers, as they were in her mother's case.

Do You Possess Behaviors the Dreamers Shared?

After reading all the stories of the women in Dr. Larry Burk's Breast Cancer Dreams Project, I made a list of the qualities and behaviors many of them shared and survived.

Many were great self-advocates, not great patients but excellent e-patients, who did research their symptoms and dreams and used the information to stay alive. They were told they had unremarkable mammograms or negative tests results and to go home, but they refused to be dismissed. They never gave up! They challenged the medical community to prove them wrong. The dreamers were asymptomatic under the definition of medical breast cancer symptoms, but their dreams were a symptom of their illness. Their dreams were early warning signs of cancer that saved their lives. Their diagnostic, healing and precognitive dreams/nightmares were all validated by accurate medical pathology reports.

You were born with a purpose, even if your parents told you that you "just happened" in the back seat of the old Ford. You accidentally happened on purpose. Your difficult journeys in life may be part of your life purpose, or soul contract, as discussed in Wanda's Chapter 37. Although we may not know our life purpose or soul mission, we have our dreams, inner guidance, and guardian angels to keep us on the right path when we come to life's fork in the road. They speak to us through the Sacred Dream Doorways.

Journaling your dreams can help you remember their guidance, and dream track, which can save your life. I understand some people cannot remember their dreams, but your inner voice speaks to you just as loudly in daydreams, prayers, and meditations, as shown in this book. Listen. With your Divine Default System, and your Celestial Army behind you, know that you are never alone in your darkest hour and miracles are a daily occurrence. Watch for the dream miracle called validation in your waking world, as in Dr. Larry's Hero's Journey dream in Chapter 52. Larry was told he would have "an exciting adventure in a creative writing assignment while on his way to see the Wizard." His precognitive dream is the reality you are reading, now. Validation!

In conclusion, this book reflects what Wanda Paulette, Denise, and I all felt: "I am alive because of my dreams."

"Further Down the Yellow Brick Road..."
— **LARRY BURK, MD, CEHP**

Kat and I have started off with you to the see the Wizard in this book, but we realize that there will be more dream adventures to come in the future. Hopefully, my breast biopsy pilot study at Duke will inspire others to do more cancer dream research in other academic centers and that there will be funding along the Yellow Brick Road to support it. In the meantime, please contact us through our websites with other stories of health-related dreams that we can include in our next books, especially if there is medical proof of the details.

APPENDICES

Appendix 1
Frequently Asked Dream Questions

Sharing dreams can be tricky. What if someone does not believe you and laughs at you? This is a genuine concern that haunted me, until I realized that it would be much easier to live with people laughing at me because I shared a dream, which did or did not come true, than crying with everyone as I am dying, because I did not share a dream that could have saved my life. When it comes to life-saving-dreams, dare to share.

1. Can we train our brain to remember our dreams? If yes, how?

Yes, we can train our brain to remember dreams, just as we can train it to wake us at a certain hour every morning or put a puzzle together. Here is how to start training your brain for sleep memory. Set your intention before you go to sleep to remember your dream when you awaken in the morning. When you do awaken, lie still, and slowly remember any emotional "snippets" of your dream. A snippet is your tiny nugget of golden information. Training yourself to remember the emotional fragments will also help you put the rest of your dream puzzle together.

2. Are early morning dreams the easiest to remember? If yes, why?

Early morning dreams are the easiest to remember because you are coming up from the REM (rapid eye movement) level of sleep through the Theta Level, and early morning dreams are the last ones you have during your sleep. The Theta Level is often used for healing. Keep a journal beside your bed, and write down your dreams in order to know if your early morning dreams come true. This gives you a way of going back to see what the dreams were or what the validation was in your waking world. In your dream state, you may travel the Time Continuum, or you may receive valuable information from your spirit guides or guardian angels. They know you may have an easier time remembering early morning dreams.

3. What does it feel like to have a dream?

It depends on the type of dream. If it is not a lucid dream, you are not aware that you are dreaming, and the dream is your reality. You feel in the dream as you would during your waking life. Just as when you are awake you do not focus on dreaming, while you are dreaming you do not focus on anything except the dream. Everything, no matter how strange, seems perfectly normal, until you wake up and remember it. Now, if you are having a lucid dream, you are aware that you are dreaming, and that makes you feel differently about your state of reality. With time and practice, you can learn to become an actively aware dreamer and change your dream. I hope this helps you.

4. Are our dreams messages to ourselves?

Yes, our dreams are very many messages to ourselves, and they can change our lives, and sometimes the lives of others we know and love. You can meet many of the inner selves that make up your total being in your dreams. You can also meet your Physician-within, to help heal yourself. In my book, I met many of my inner selves, including a mentally challenged boy named Billy who regularly turned up in my dreams to give me guidance. And he was fantastic.

5. Can I talk to past relatives in a dream? If yes, how?

Absolutely! Sometimes it is as easy as voicing your request before you go to sleep at night. This is known as setting your dream intention (see Part Four).Remember, in the dream world of the Time Continuum discussed by Einstein in his theories, there is no past or future; everything is NOW. The universe is always listening and has the "direct phone number" for our deceased loved ones.

Make sure you write your dreams down, because it can be hard to recognize our dead loved ones as they often return to their "prime body form," how they appeared when they were in their prime or at their most healthy. They may be young again, for example, making it difficult to recognize them. They may only speak with you for a few seconds. Before I even knew I had breast cancer, I had a prophetic dream in which my deceased mother came into my dream looking very healthy and younger, took my hands and said, "You are going to be just fine." I woke up wondering what she meant by that, because I was not aware anything was wrong with me. Months later, I began to have the breast cancer nightmares, then I got the pathology report diagnosis. During treatment and many other times afterwards, I would have a deceased loved one "pop" into dreams and hold a conversation with me. Sometimes I would recognize them, and sometimes they would look so young and different it was not until I awoke and remembered something they said (that rang a bell) that I recognized them, which was also a validation of their identity. When I would find their picture in an album, I would remember them from the dream in their younger healthy state of life.

Appendix 2
Glossary of Dream Terminology

ACTIVE LUCID DREAMS - You know you are dreaming while dreaming by being aware of the environment in the dream and actively participating in the dream.

AWAKE DREAM - the transitional state from wakefulness to sleep, or sleep to wakefulness known as hypnagogia, a hypnogogic state of consciousness, or threshold consciousness. Although the dreamer may be awake, their dream may continue. An awake dream can include lucid thought, lucid dreaming, hallucinations, and sleep paralysis.

CONSCIOUSNESS - level of alertness.

DAYDREAM - transient lapses in the control of attention focused on your external world that can lead to a shift in attention similar to meditation, prayer, or self-vocalization.

DREAM ARCHETYPES - dream symbols that possess the same universal meaning for all men and women.

Dream Incubation - to "plant a seed" in the mind for a specific dream topic to occur, either for health, wealth, love, recreation, or to attempt to solve a problem.

DREAM JOURNAL - A dream diary in which dream experiences are recorded and used for dream tracking.

DREAM JOURNALING - the act of recording dreams and dream experiences in some fashion, such as in a written diary, spoken recording, or artwork.

DREAM REENTRY - the act of slipping back into a specific dream from a waking state.

DREAM SPIRIT GUIDE - an entity in dreams that remains a disincarnate spirit in order to act as a guide or protector to a living human dreamer. Spirit guides can take many forms.

DREAM SUBCATEGORIES - a dream subordinate category or a division of a category.

DREAMS THAT COME TRUE - see precognitive dreams.

DREAM TRACKING - keeping track of dreams that may be recurrent or significant through journaling.

DREAM TRACKING - using dream journaling to track messages in dreams to track information and watch for dream validation.

DUALITY - two elements in a dream that have a concealed form in symbolism and a revealed form in the obvious.

DÉJÀ VU - an expression used to describe an intuitive experience that seems to spark our memory of a place, person, or experience we have already seen or done. The expression is derived from the French, meaning "already seen."

EPIC DREAMS - many dreams at once but always big in nature; also referred to as great dreams, cosmic dreams, or numinous dreams. Dreams so huge, compelling, and vivid they cannot be ignored.

GUIDED DREAMS - dreams in which human spirit guides or animal guides share information for healing or personal growth. They are often shamanic in nature. (See shamanic dreams.)

GUIDED IMAGERY - the use of words, music, or pictures, or all three, to evoke imagery or imaginary scenarios in a subject to bring about some beneficial or desired effect.

HEALING DREAMS - teach you something significant about yourself or someone else and are further call-to-action dreams to make a change in your life.

HYPNAGOGIC STATE OF CONSCIOUSNESS - See awake dream.

INFORMATIVE DREAM - different from a diagnostic dream, in that it shares information that can be current or precognitive.

INNER VOICE - internal monologue, internal speech, verbal stream of consciousness, thinking in words

LITERAL - a first-person view of the dream in literal detail. The message in the dream is crystal clear upon awakening.

LUCID DREAM - you know you are dreaming while dreaming.

MEDITATION - also a form of lucid daydreaming.

NIGHTMARES - a frightening or unpleasant dream, sometimes referred to as night terrors.

PRECOGNITIVE DREAMS – also known as prophetic dreams, psychic dreams, primordial dreams, divination dreams, premonition dreams, guided dreams, shamanic dreams, and dreams that come true.

PROPHETIC DREAMS - also known as psychic dreams, primordial dreams, divination dreams, premonition dreams, and dreams that come true, and can be validated by facts, scientific tests, or life events.

RECURRENT DREAMS – dreams that are experienced repeatedly over a long or short period of time. They can be pleasant or nightmarish and are unique to the person and their experiences. They are recurrent because the dreamer has not resolved an issue, making them a dream call to action.

REM - **r**apid **e**ye **m**ovement seen during sleep.

SACRED DREAM DOORS - doorways to a parallel universe where passed-over loved ones, guardian angels, and spirit guides can speak with you.

SHAMANIC DREAMS – are the sister to healing dreams, dream journeys in which the dreamer often flies to new places in order to access knowledge, request healing, meet power animals and healing guides, find power plants, or conduct soul retrievals. Shamanic dreams often have the power of the number three in them.

SLEEPING - an altered state of alertness.

SYMBOLIC - signs, symbols and abstract information that may not be understood or realized until the actual event takes place later in the waking world.

TANDEM DREAMING - when dreamers share or enter each other's dreams simultaneously during the night.

TRANSCENDING - to be, outdo, or go beyond the range or limits of something abstract, or to surpass in excellence, elevation, and excel

UNCONSCIOUSNESS - the part of the mind inaccessible to the conscious mind that affects behavior and emotions. It is synonyms with subconscious, psyche, id, ego, super-ego, and inner-self.

UNIVERSAL CONSCIOUSNESS - aka Universal Google or Universal Oneness, a concept that embraces the underlying idea that the essence of all being and becoming is connected to the universe.

Appendix 3
Glossary of Medical Terminology

COMPUTED TOMOGRAPHY (CT) - produces cross-sectional images of the body using ionizing radiation and optional iodine contrast agents

MAMMOGRAPHY - uses conventional radiographs with ionizing radiation and compression to examine the breasts

MAGNETIC RESONANCE IMAGING (MRI) – produces cross-sectional images of the body using magnetic fields and non-ionizing radio frequencies with optional gadolinium contrast agents

THERMOGRAPHY - produces images of the body by detecting infrared heat from the skin surface without any form of radiation

ULTRASOUND - produces cross-sectional images of the body using non-ionizing sound waves from hand-held probes

Endnotes

Preface

1. Bronkhorst, A.W. The cocktail party phenomenon: A review of research on speech intelligibility in multiple-talker conditions. Acta Acustica united with Acustica. 2000;86:117–128. Retrieved April 18, 2010.

2 Newman, R. S. The cocktail party effect in infants revisited: Listening to one's name in noise. Developmental Psychology. 2005;41 (2):352–362.

3 Wood N. and Cowan N. The cocktail party phenomenon revisited: How frequent are attention shifts to one's name in an irrelevant auditory channel? J Exp Psychol Learn Mem Cogn. 1995;21 (1): 255-60. PMID 7876773. doi:10.1037/0278-7393.21.1.255.

4 Barrat, E. and Davis, N. Autonomous Sensory Meridian Response (ASMR): a flow-like mental state. Peer J. 2015;3: e851. PMC 4380153. PMID 25834771. doi:10.7717/peerj.851.

5 Mitchell, J. Latest social media craze: Autonomous Sensory Meridian Response. The Maine Public Broadcasting Network. September 2, 2012. Retrieved January 20, 2016.

Introduction: The History of Healing Dreams

6 Krippner, S. Humanity's first healers: Psychological and psychiatric stances on shamans and shamanism. Rev Psiq Clín. 2007;34S(1):16-22.

7 Harner, M. J. The Way of the Shaman (San Francisco: Harper & Row, 1990), pp. 99.

8 Genacarelle, S and Reina, R. A Man Among the Helpers (Virtualbookworm. com Publishing, 2012).

9 Mails, T. E. and Chief Eagle, D. Fools Crow: Wisdom and Power (Tulsa, OK: Council Oaks Books, 1991), pp.74.

10 Sigerist, H. E. A History of Medicine Volume 2: Early Greek, Hindu, and Persian Medicine (1st ed.). (New York: Oxford University Press, 1987), pp. 63.

11 Wilcox, R. A. and Whitham, E. M. The symbol of modern medicine: Why one snake is more than two. Ann Intern Med. 2003;138(8):673-677. doi:10.7326/0003-4819-138-8-200304150-00016.

12 Schredl, M. Freud's interpretation of his own dreams in The Interpretation of Dreams: A continuity hypothesis perspective. Int J Dream Research. 2008;1(2):44-47.

13 Hersh, T. How might we explain the parallels between Freud's 1895 Irma dream and his 1923 cancer? Dreaming. 1995;5(4):267-287.

14 Jung, C. G. Collected Works, The Practice of Psychotherapy, 2nd Ed. (London: Routledge & Kegan Paul, 1966) Vol 16, pp.73.

15 Jung, C. G. Collected Works, The Structure and Dynamics of the Psyche (2nd ed.), (London: Routledge & Kegan Paul, 1969) Vol 8, pp. 290.

16 Lazarus, J. Dreams: Listening to the Voice of God. (Durham, NC: Welkin Books; 1st edition, 2011).

17 Edgar Cayce Readings, (Virginia Beach, VA: Association for Research and Enlightenment), pp. 136-7.

18 Edgar Cayce Readings, (Virginia Beach, VA: Association for Research and Enlightenment), pp. 1537-1.

19 Kasatkin, V. N. Teoriya Snovidenii (Theory of Dreams) (Leningrad: Meditsina, 1967), pp. 352.

20 Van de Castle, R. L. Our Dreaming Mind (New York: Ballantine Books, 1994), pp. 362-364.

21 Kasatkin, V. translated by Susanne van Doorn, A Theory of Dreams (Lulu. com, 2014), pp. 16, 17.

22 Royston, R. and Humphries, A. The Hidden Power of Dreams: A Guide to Understanding Their Meaning. (London: Bantam Books, 2006).

23 Barasch, M. I. Healing Dreams: Exploring the Dreams that Can Transform Your Life. (New York: Riverhead Books, 2000), pp. 66-88.

24 Burk, L. Let Magic Happen: Adventures in Healing with a Holistic Radiologist (Durham, NC: Healing Imager Press, 2012), pp. 316-318.

1 Origins of the Breast Cancer Dreams Project

25 Burk, L. Warning dreams preceding the diagnosis of breast cancer: a survey of the most important characteristics. Explore. 2015; 11(3), 193–198.

26 Krippner, S., and Ullman, M. Telepathy and dreams: A controlled experiment with electroencephalogram-electro-oculogram monitoring. Journal of Nervous and Mental Disease. 1970;51:394-403.

27 Lee-Shield, S. My appeal. July 4, 2013. http://soniaslifeappeal.wordpress.com/myappeal/

28 Burch W.E. She Who Dreams: A Journey into Healing Through Dream-work (Novato, CA: New World Library, 2003).

29 Burk L. Prodromal dreams of breast cancer and clinical correlation. Presentation at the IASD PsiberDreaming Conference, 2013. http://www. letmagichappen.com/images/uploads/documents/pdc2013-burk.Breast-CancerDreams.pdf.

30 Dossey, L. One Mind: How Our Individual Mind Is Part of a Greater Consciousness and Why It Matters. (Carlsbad, CA: Hay House Inc, 2013).

31 Kinney, C.K. Transcending breast cancer: reconstructing one's self. Issues in Mental Health Nursing. 1996;17:201-216.

2   A Feather for Your Dreams

32 Burk, L. Warning dreams preceding the diagnosis of breast cancer: a survey of the most important characteristics. Explore. 2015;11(3):193–198.

33 DreamsCloud https://www.dreamscloud.com

34 Dr. Oz Show: The Sixth Sense: Shocking Premonitions with Kathleen O'Keefe-Kanavos (2, 2017; NY, NY.)

35 Kanavos, Kathleen O'Keefe: Surviving Cancerland: Intuitive Aspects of Healing (Fort Bragg, CA: Cypress House, 2014), pp. 4-27.

3   Warning Dreams Preceding the Diagnosis of Breast Cancer Research Results

36 Burk, L. Warning dreams preceding the diagnosis of breast cancer: a survey of the most important characteristics. Explore. 2015;11(3):193–198.

37 Zackrisson, S., Andersson, I., Janzon, L., Manjer, J., Garne, J.P.: Rate of over-diagnosis of breast cancer 15 years after end of Malmö mammographic screening trial: follow-up study. BMJ. 2006;332(7543):689–692.

38 BRCA1 and BRCA2: Cancer risk and genetic testing. http://www.cancer. gov/cancertopics/causes-prevention/genetics/brca-fact-sheet#r27.

39 Shiovitz, S. and Korde, L.A. Genetics of breast cancer: a topic in evolution. Ann. Oncol. 2015;26(7): 1291–1299.

40 SEER Stat Fact Sheets: Breast Cancer. http://seer.cancer.gov/statfacts/ html/breast.html.

41 Biller-Andorno, N. and Juni, P. Abolishing mammography screening programs? A view from the Swiss Medical Board. NEJM. 2014;370(21):1965-7. doi: 10.1056/NEJMp1401875. Epub 2014 Apr 16.

42 U.S. Preventive Services Task Force. Screening for Breast Cancer: U.S. Preventive Services Task Force recommendation statement. Ann. Intern. Med. 2009;151(10):716–726, W-236.

43 Mainiero, M.B., et al. ACR appropriateness criteria breast cancer screening. J. Am. Coll. Radiol. 2013;10(1):11–14.

44 Berg, W., Kuhl, C.K., et al. Mammography, breast ultrasound, and magnetic resonance imaging for surveillance of women at high familial risk for breast cancer. JCO. 2005;23(33):8469–8476.

45 Corsetti, V., Houssami, N., Ferrari, A., et al. Breast screening with ultra-sound in women with mammography-negative dense breasts: evidence on incremental cancer detection and false positives, and associated cost. Eur. J. Cancer. 2008;44:539–544.

46 Hudson, T. Journey to Hope: Leaving the Fear of Breast Cancer Behind. (Naples, FL: Brush and Quill Productions, 2011).

4   The Rise of the Dreaming E-Patient

47 Published in the Austin American-Statesman from 4/19/2006 - 4/22/2006

5   Basic Dream Categories

48 Buckner, R. L., Andrews-Hanna, J. R., and Schacter, D. L. The brain's default network: anatomy, function, and relevance to disease. Annals of the New York Academy of Science. 2008;1124:1-38. doi: 10.1196/annals.1440.011

49 Psychology Today: July 30, 2011, Patrick McNamara, PhD.

50 http://besthealthus.com/wellness/sleep/nightmare-causes/http://www.sleepeducation.org/sleep-disorders-by-category/parasomnias/nightmares/overview American Academy of Sleep Medicine.

51 Waggoner, R. Lucid Dreaming: The Gateway to the Inner Self. (Needham, MA: Moment Point Press, 2008).

12 Transcending Breast Cancer: Reconstructing One's Self

52 Singer, J. Seeing Through the Visible World: Jung, Gnosis, and Chaos. (New York: Harper Collins, 1990).

14 "Three Crabs, Three Pearls, and a Physician-within"

53 Kanovos, Kathleen O'Keefe. Surviving Cancerland: Intuitive Aspects of Healing. Chapter 25: "Doctor Within, Heal Thyself." (Fort Bragg, CA: Cypress House, 2014), pp. 140-142.

Benign and Malignant Brain Tumors Medical Introduction (Featuring Mark Ruffalo's Dream Cancer Story.)

54 A dream that led Mark Ruffalo to discover he had a brain tumor. Flip the Movie Script, March 8, 2016, http://flipthemoviescript.com/dream-led-mark-ruffalo-discover-brain-tumor/.

22 "Go for an X-ray"

55 Helvie, C. You Can Beat Lung Cancer: Using Alternative/Integrative Interventions. (Winchester, UK: Ayni Books, 2012).

26 The Rape

56 Hagood, L. Awakening to dreams. Journal of Religion and Health. 2006;45(2):160-170.

28 Dead Sucking Insects

57 Delevitt, P. Wyld Possibilities. (Charlottesville, NC: Wyld Possibilities Press, 1999), pp.30.

30 Ways to Remember Your Dreams

58 Boodman, S. Doctors' diagnostic errors are often not mentioned but can take a serious toll. Kaiser Health News, May 6, 2013.

59 Dreams. (n.d.). In International Association for the Study of Dreams. Retrieved June 30, 2015, from http://www.asdreams.org/aboutdreams/

60 Graduate Studies in Dreams and Dreaming. (n.d.). In International Association for the Study of Dreams.

61 American Institute of Physics. Baby's first dreams: Sleep cycles of the fetus. ScienceDaily. April 14, 2009. www.sciencedaily.com/releases/2009/04/090413185734.htm.

38 Tiny Bubbles and Fishy Chakras

62 Waggoner, R. Lucid Dreaming: Gateway to the Inner Self. (Needham, MA: Moment Point Press, 2008).

39 The Raw Food Diet Dream

63 Burk, L. Let Magic Happen: Adventures in Healing with a Holistic Radiologist (Durham, NC: Healing Imager Press, 2012), pp.136.

41 Bliss behind the Mask of Addiction

64 Morse, M. and Perry, P. Transformed by the Light: The Powerful Effect of Near-Death Experiences on People's Lives (New York: Villard Books, 1992).

46 Cancer or Not Cancer?

65 http://www.telegraph.co.uk/news/science/science-news/3353504/Black-and-white-TV-generation-have-monochrome-dreams.html

66 Burk, L. Psychic/intuitive diagnosis: Two case reports and commentary. JAltern Complement Med [letter] 1997;3(3):209-11.

51 "Your Cables are Twisted"

67 Fishman L, Dombi G, Michealsen C, et al. Piriformis syndrome: Diagnosis, treatment, and outcome. A 10-year study. Arch Phys Med Rehabil. 2002;83:295-301.

68 Pace, J. B. and Nagle, D. Piriformis syndrome. Western J. Med. 1976;124: 4359.

69 Benson E. R. and Schutzer, S. F. Posttraumatic piriformis syndrome: diagnosis and results of operative treatment. JBJS. 1999;81(7):941-9.

52 The Hero's Journey into the Underworld

70 Campbell, J. The Hero with a Thousand Faces. (Princeton, NJ: Princeton University Press, 2004).

Additional Reading

Burk, Larry, MD, CEHP. *Let Magic Happen: Adventures in Healing with a Holistic Radiologist.* Durham, NC: Healing Imager Press, 2012.

Burch, Wanda. *She Who Dreams: A Journey into Healing through Dreamwork.* San Francisco, CA: New World Library, 2003.

Kemper, Kathi J. MD, MPH. *Authentic Healing: A Practical Guide for Caregivers.* Minneapolis, MN: Two Harbors Press, 2016.

Newmark, Amy and Kelly Sullivan Walden. *Chicken Soup for the Soul: Dreams and Premonitions: 101 Amazing Stories of Miracles, Divine Intervention, and Insight.* Cos Cob, CT: Chicken Soup for the Soul, 2015.

O' Brien, Deborah. *Bliss: Behind the Mask.* Carlsbad, CA: Balboa Press, a division of Hay House, 2015.

O'Keefe-Kanavos, Kathleen. *Surviving Cancerland: Intuitive Aspects of Healing.* Cypress House, Fort Bragg, CA, 2014.

Siegel, Bernie S., MD. *A Book of Miracles: Inspiring True Stories of Healing, Gratitude, and Love.* Reprint. San Francisco, CA: New World Library, 2014.

_____. *Love, Medicine and Miracles: Lessons Learned about Self-Healing from a Surgeon's Experience with Exceptional Patients.* Reprint. New York: William Morrow, 2011.

Van de Castle, Robert L. *Our Dreaming Mind.* New York: Ballantine Books, 1994.

Walden, Kelly Sullivan. *It's All in Your Dreams: Five Portals to an Awakened Life.* Newbury Port, MA: Conari Press, an imprint of Red Wheel/Weiser, 2013.

Biographies of Contributors

LARRY BURK, MD, CEHP., President of Healing Imager, PC, in Durham, NC, specializes in teleradiology, Emotional Freedom Techniques (EFT), hypnosis, and dreamwork. He was one of the pioneering researchers in MRI of the knee and shoulder. He later trained in acupuncture and hypnosis and is a Certified Energy Health Practitioner. He was a co-founder of Duke Integrative Medicine and is now a consulting associate in radiology at Duke University Medical Center.

He also maintains a part-time coaching practice at Oriental Health Solutions, LLC. Dr. Burk is a Medical Intuition and Symbolic Healing guest trainer at the Monroe Institute. He is a founding member of the American Board of Scientific Medical Intuition, a member of the International Association for the Study of Dreams, and a former board president of the Rhine Research Center. His book, *Let Magic Happen: Adventures in Healing with a Holistic Radiologist,* was published in 2012. He gave a TEDx talk on "Cancer Warning Dreams that Can Save Your Life" in March 2016.

Links for his talk, papers, blogs, and newsletters can be found at *www.larry burkmd.com.*

KATHLEEN (KAT) O'KEEFE-KANAVOS is a three-time cancer survivor whose guided dreams diagnosed her illness, as seen on *The Dr. Oz Show*, NBC News, American Express Open, and in newspapers and magazines and detailed in her multi-award winning book, *Surviving Cancerland*, along with *Chicken Soup for the Soul: Dreams and Premonitions.* Kat taught Special Education in Florida's Lee County Schools, wrote curriculum, and taught psychology at University of Southern Florida, Fort Myers Branch. Kat is an author, lecturer, and TV/radio host and producer. She is producer of *Wicked Housewives On Cape Cod,* host of the *Kat Kanavos Show* on New Earth TV, an internationally syndicated columnist for *Women's Voices Magazine* and BizCatalyst360, and lectures on patient advocacy and spiritual guidance.

For more information, log on to *www.KathleenOkeefeKanavos.com.*

KATHI KEMPER MD, MPH is the founding director of the Center for Integrative Health and Wellness; a professor of Pediatrics at Ohio State University; has served on the faculty of the Universities of Washington, Yale, and Harvard; and has founded three academic Centers for Integrative Medicine in Boston, North Carolina, and Ohio.

She has published over 170 peer-reviewed research papers and four books for the general public. She is past president of the Academic Pediatric Association, founded the American Academy of Pediatrics Section on Integrative Medicine, and serves as editor-in-chief of the international journal, *Complementary Therapies in Medicine*. Her most recent book published in 2016 is *Authentic Healing: A Practical Guide for Caregivers*.

Dr. Kemper is recognized internationally as the founder of the field of Integrative Pediatrics and is frequently consulted by media, including the New York Times, Chicago Tribune, Newsweek, ABC News, the Wall Street Journal, Redbook, and USA Today.

SAVITRI SIMPSON is the author of multiple books, including *The Meaning of Dreaming*. She has a Bachelor of Arts Degree from the University of Waco, Texas. Savitri lives with her husband, Sudarshan, in a dome home at Ananda Village, a cooperative spiritual community in Northern California, guided by the teaching of Paramhansa Yogananda and founded by Swami Kriyananda. She is a member of the Nayaswami Order, so she is called Nayaswami Savitri

For more information, log on to *www.savitrisimpson.com*.

ROCIO AGUIRRE is a certified coach, transformational educator, and speaker who has worked in the corporate world for 20 years in technology and professional development, both in the learning industry. She helps people achieve their full potential and find meaning in their lives through the use of dreamwork, mindfulness, and other modalities. She is founder of *Awake and Live Your Dreams*.

For more information, log on to *www.magloireaguirre.com*.

ATHENA KOLINSKI, MA is a Religious Studies professor at the University of Philosophical Research, where she obtained her second master's degree in Consciousness Studies. She also received an M.A. and B.A. from California State University, Northridge. Athena is a certified Tarotpy practitioner, a New Dreamwork coach, and 2017–18 Logistics Lead for the International Association for the Study of Dreams.

For more information, log on to *www.starcarddreaming.com*.

REBECCA GERACITANO is a certified hypnotherapist located in Louisville, Kentucky. Having had her first past-life awareness at the young age of six and then later past-life dreams, her own journey with reincarnation and regression has inspired her to help others on their spiritual path to wholeness.

For more information, log on to *www.integrativemind.net.*

DEBORAH O'BRIEN, author of *Bliss: Behind the Mask*, is an inspirational speaker, meditation teacher, spiritual life coach, and self-image consultant. Twenty-six years ago, during a near-death experience and healing dream encounter, she experienced a spiritual awakening. She now teaches the same eight-stage process that healed her life that day as tools to liberate women from destructive patterns and limiting beliefs.

For more information, log on to *www.deborahobrienbliss.com.*

INKA NISINBAUM had a double lung and liver transplant in 2002, due to cystic fibrosis. She has a master's degree in psychology; is a published author in Germany, where she's originally from; and is a motivational speaker. Inka is the only woman worldwide who had a baby after her kind of transplant.

For more information, log on to *www.inkanisinbaum.com.*

MARIA MARS became a Beautiful Dreamer at age 10, when she learned to play the song on her electric organ. She has documented sleeping and waking dreams for over two decades, explores the multidimensional messages of the cosmic conscious dreamer, and facilitates conscious transformational experiences, aka The Art of Ourselves (TAO). Maria is a quality specialist, conscious barefoot dancer, tree-hugger, writer, and artist.

PATRICIA ROSE UPCZAK is an author, reiki master, workshop leader, and teacher. She lives in the Rocky Mountains. She is currently working on several new books and a *Creativity, Thinking, and Education* podcast launch.

For more information, go to *www.HappyTeachersHappyStudents.com.*

CAROLYN K. KINNEY, PhD, RN, a retired nursing professor, served on the Schools of Nursing faculty at the Universities of Iowa, Michigan, and Texas (Austin and Galveston). Dr. Kinney devoted her nursing career to integrating holistic healing perspectives into mainstream healthcare. She also offered individual, family, and group counseling services based on the modeling and role-modeling nursing theory.

PAULETTE WYSSBROD-GOLTZ has just finished a BS in Psychology and is a freelance writer for three online platforms. She left Corporate America after a bout with breast cancer and her writing passion became stronger than ever. *Bully*, her first completed novel, came about during NANOWRIMO (National Novel Writing Month, November 2015). Writing, reading, music, and movies now consume her waking hours. She currently resides in Lake Jackson, Texas with her family.

For more information, log on to *https://pwgwrites.com*.

WANDA BURCH is a 26-year breast cancer survivor. In 2003, New World Library published the story of her experience of healing and dreams: *She Who Dreams: A Journey into Healing through Dreamwork*. As a retired historian, she works in historic preservation and on boards of historic societies and museums. She continues to work with dreams and with breast cancer advocacy programs.

Information about her books can be found at *www.wandaburch.com*.

SUZANNE M. DE GREGORIO was raised in southern New Jersey and graduated from the University of Kentucky with a degree in Political Science and a field of concentration in International Relations. She is a grassroots advocate for autism, environmental issues, and the legalization of medical cannabis. Suzanne runs a food pantry for a community ministry in east Louisville. She lives with her husband and son in Louisville, Kentucky.

Her blog is *http://moonbeamsecodreams.blogspot.com*.

DANA WALDEN is former chairman of the Education Commission for IREO (Intergovernmental Renewable Energy Organization), founding board member of Fostering a Change (housing and program support for women aging out of the foster care system), and co-founder of The Dream Project (empowerment program for youth), as well as an internationally acclaimed composer, performer, producer, and director. His Muse Management approach is dedicated to "the dream realized." He is director of Strategic Insights and Creative Implementation for CHIME IN (the Change Is Me International).

For more information, log on to *www.LuvHubProductions.com*.

DANA LYNNE ANDERSEN, MA is a visionary multimedia artist, writer, and vehicle for transformation who has taught and exhibited on three continents. She founded *Awakening Arts Academy,* which has centers at the Ananda Laurelwood Campus in Portland, Oregon, and Ananda Europa in Assisi, Italy. She offers courses and certification in Transformative Arts. Her work has been featured in newspapers, radio, television, and on the covers of books and magazines.

For more information, log on to *http://danalynneandersen.com.*

JANE KATRA, PhD taught Public Health at the University of Oregon. She has provided manysuccessful results in several psychic research studies, and has also practiced as a spiritual healer for 42 years. She experienced a very high vibrational domain in an NDE in 1994 where she was instructed to activate others' subtle energy systems. She also experiences after-death communications in the waking and dream states. Dr. Katra is the co-author of two books with physicist Russell Targ: *The Heart of the Mind: Using Our Mind to Transform Our Consciousness*, and *Miracles of Mind: Exploring Nonlocal Consciousness and Spiritual Healing.*

For more information, log on to *www.janekatra.org.*

Enhance Your Book Club

Dreams That Can Save Your Life: Early Warning Signs of Cancer and Other Illnesses offers numerous complexities that require differing points of view, such as:

1. Medical science versus dream intuition and conventional therapy versus holistic therapy.

2. Can dreams used as a diagnostic tool and medical testing for early diagnosis of health conditions coexist and be complementary or only be antagonistic to conventional medicine?

3. Discuss which dream stories had the greatest impact on you and why.

4. Discuss ways in which a person can use dreams to self-advocate to avoid being a victim of circumstance.

5. Discuss your feelings about spirit guides, angels, voices, and gut instincts, or intuition.

Also of interest from Findhorn Press

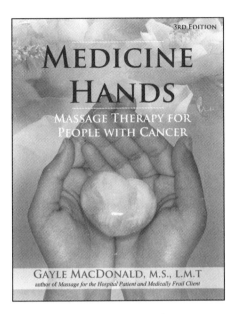

Medicine Hands
by Gayle MacDonald

THE FIELD OF ONCOLOGY massage is maturing into a discipline with a deeper and deeper body of knowledge. The 3rd edition of *Medicine Hands* reflects this maturation. Every chapter contains updated information and insights into massaging people affected by cancer.

New chapters have been added to cover each stage of the cancer experience: treatment, recovery, survivorship, side effects from the disease, and end of life. These new chapters and organizational structure will make it easier for the reader to find the information needed to plan the massage session for a given client. In addition, a new chapter has been added that focuses on the Pressure/ Site/Positioning framework. This is the clinical framework around which the massage session is planned.

978-1-84409-639-8

FINDHORN PRESS

Life-Changing Books

Learn more about us and our books at
www.findhornpress.com

For information on the Findhorn Foundation:
www.findhorn.org

PLEASE SEND US THIS CARD TO RECEIVE OUR LATEST CATALOG FREE OF CHARGE.

Book in which this card was found _____

☐ Check here to receive our catalog via e-mail.

Company _____

☐ Send me wholesale information

Name _____

Address _____ Phone _____

City _____ State _____ Zip _____ Country _____

E-mail address _____

Please check area(s) of interest to receive related announcements via e-mail:

☐ Health   ☐ Self-help   ☐ Science/Nature   ☐ Shamanism

☐ Ancient Mysteries   ☐ New Age/Spirituality   ☐ Visionary Plants   ☐ Martial Arts

☐ Spanish Language   ☐ Sexuality/Tantra   ☐ Family and Youth   ☐ Religion/Philosophy

Please send a catalog to my friend:

Name _____ Company _____

Address _____ Phone _____

City _____ State _____ Zip _____ Country _____

Order at 1-800-246-8648 • Fax (802) 767-3726

E-mail: customerservice@InnerTraditions.com • Web site: www.InnerTraditions.com

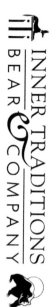

Inner Traditions • Bear&Company

P.O. Box 388

Rochester, VT 05767-0388

U.S.A.